Lab Values

Everything You Need to Know about Laboratory Medicine and its Importance in the Diagnosis of Diseases

DAVID ANDERSSON

First edition   20

CONTENTS

1. INTRODUCTION

The need for medical students to familiarize themselves with laboratory medicine is evident. It is said that approximately 60-70% of decision making in medicine is done based on the results of laboratory tests. Laboratory values essentially provide data in an objective form that relates to the patient's health. They can aid in early diagnosis of diseases that have not yet had clinical manifestations, thereby leading to more effective management of such conditions. They can also aid in monitoring the progress of various diseases so that treatment can be modified accordingly.

Despite the facts stated above, laboratory medicine remains a highly underrated area in the field of medicine. The Centers for Disease Control (2008) stated that insufficient understanding of laboratory tests in a clinical setting can lead to misinterpretation of results, which may jeopardize patient safety. They also stated that inefficient test selection could increase healthcare costs. This book aims at helping medical students differentiate between normal and abnormal laboratory results. It also helps them place these in proper clinical context.

While interpreting the laboratory values is basically the job of the primary healthcare provider, that is, the physician, a basic knowledge in this area is essential for nurses, in order to recognize trends that can affect patients, which would in turn help in framing a good healthcare plan. Since laboratory medicine is a key area in patient care, there is a separate section on laboratory values alone in tests such as the NCLEX. This is an area which most nurses find difficult, as you're expected to memorize a range of numbers that present normal values. A nurse appearing for NCLEX must also know how to properly obtain blood specimens from a peripheral or central line. Nurses must not only be able to detect if a certain laboratory value is abnormal, but must also be in a position to explain to the patient the need for such tests and the exact procedure that would be followed. They should also be able to advise patients on how to prepare for the test, as, for example, if fasting for a certain period is required. Nurses also play a key role in monitoring the laboratory values of patients with existing diseases. Most importantly, they should be aware of whether or not the laboratory results warrant urgent communication with the primary healthcare provider.

For easy understanding, this book has been categorized into various sections based on the similarity of laboratory tests that are to be performed. The last section deals with grouping of tests that are done routinely, in emergencies, or in special healthcare situations. Various tables have been designed for ease of memorization. At the end of the book, there is an exercise section which contains multiple choice questions. The answers are detailed at the end of the book.

This book is by no means an exhaustive report and does not cover all of the laboratory tests that are done in several healthcare facilities. During routine practice, you may need to keep a laboratory manual handy. It is also worthwhile remembering that the term 'normal' varies from facility to facility and different laboratories may have a different range of values. This book gives normal values that have been sourced from standard references. However, minor variations in day-to-day practice are possible.

2. OBTAINING LABORATORY SAMPLES-THE CORRECT METHODS

The healthcare provider uses lab values to diagnose a patient's health condition, and assess how much medication will be useful. The laboratory values essentially measure the biochemical processes that are taking place within the patient. Therefore, in order to avoid errors, the nurse or technician must be proficient in drawing blood for lab work. The collection of a laboratory specimen in the correct manner is crucial to efficient diagnosis and treatment. This is essential to avoid possible health risks to the staff handling the specimen, and also to ensure that there are no errors in laboratory values due to incorrect collection and handling of the specimen.

TYPES OF LABORATORY SAMPLES:

It is virtually possible to test anything that has been isolated from the patient's body. A list of sources used as laboratory samples are outlined in Box 1. The more common ones have been elaborated on below.

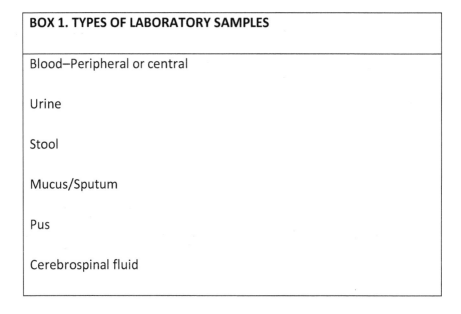

BOX 1. TYPES OF LABORATORY SAMPLES
Blood–Peripheral or central
Urine
Stool
Mucus/Sputum
Pus
Cerebrospinal fluid

PREPARING TO OBTAIN THE SAMPLE: PRIOR PREPARATION

Certain procedures must be followed prior to sampling, in order to avoid errors.

- The patient for whom the testing is done must be identified correctly, either by asking the patient or verifying their name against the patient tag.

- Specimen containers must be properly labeled with the patients' name and admission number.
- The source and quantity of specimen must be determined. Large samples of blood are best obtained using evacuated blood tube systems.
- If any prior preparation, such as fasting, was required, this must be verified with the patient prior to obtaining the specimen.

OBTAINING A BLOOD SAMPLE:

There are various kinds of blood that can be sent for laboratory tests. These are shown in Box 2 below.

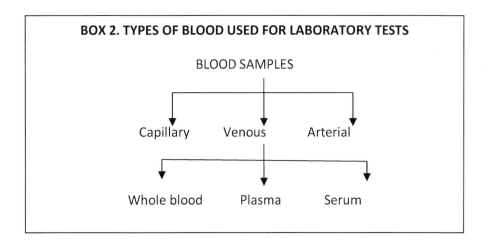

BOX 2. TYPES OF BLOOD USED FOR LABORATORY TESTS

BLOOD SAMPLES

Capillary   Venous   Arterial

Whole blood   Plasma   Serum

Venous samples:

These must be drawn using an intravenous needle. The needles may be direct ones or of butterfly type, which are generally used in smaller veins.

- A suitable vein is selected for collecting the sample. This is usually from the patient's forearm. The vein must be palpated to check its thickness.
- A tourniquet is applied on the patient's arm, a few inches above the selected donor site.
- The area is prepared using an alcohol swab and allowed to air dry.
- The patient is asked to make a fist, and the skin is stretched taut over the vein.
- The needle is inserted into the vein at a 15 to 30 degree angle.
- The blood is collected into the syringe or vacutainer tube.
- After the blood has been collected in all the tubes, the tourniquet can be taken off and the needle can be taken out.
- A gauze pad is then applied over the puncture site until the blood flow stops.
- The tubes are labeled, and any waste material is then discarded

Capillary blood:

This is a common method used for home testing, particularly in diabetic patients for monitoring blood glucose levels. It may be done using a finger stick or heel stick.

Finger stick:

- This is usually done on the middle or ring finger.
- The center of the finger, which generally has softer tissue, is used.
- The finger is first massaged and then punctured using a sterile lancet.
- The first drop is generally discarded as it contains tissue fluid.
- The blood is collected onto a collection device or tube, by applying gentle pressure on the punctured area. The finger must not be 'milked'.
- A gauze pad is then applied over the puncture site until the blood flow stops.
- The tubes are labeled, and any waste material is then discarded.

Heel stick:

- This is recommended for newborn babies.
- The heel is warmed for three minutes.
- A sterile lancet is then used to puncture the side of the heel.
- As with the finger, the first drop of blood is wiped away and the rest is collected in the micro container.
- The heel is raised and gentle pressure is applied with gauze until the blood flow stops.
- The tubes are labeled, and any waste material is then discarded.

Arterial blood:

- This is slightly more technique-sensitive than drawing venous blood, because it is usually drawn under emergency conditions. However, since these vessels pulsate, they are easier t locate.

- ABG can be drawn from the radial, brachial or femoral artery. The preparation is similar to that of a venipuncture; however, it is important to use a syringe that contains heparin to prevent coagulation. The artery is located and held between fingers of the opposite hand.

- The vessel is entered at an angle of 30 to 60 degrees for radial and brachial arteries, or at 60 to 90 degrees for the femoral artery.

- Once the arterial wall is entered, the blood will enter the syringe in a pulsatile fashion.

- Once the syringe has filled, it may be withdrawn and a gauze pressure pack must be applied for at least five minutes to stop the bleeding, and up to 30 minutes if a femoral artery was used.

- The syringe must be packed in ice and sent to the laboratory immediately. The sample must be analyzed within ten minutes for accurate results.

- After an arterial blood draw, the site must be monitored frequently for signs of hematoma, pain, or vascular compromise.

OBTAINING A URINE SAMPLE:

- If the patient has not been catheterized, a clean container must be provided to the patient for obtaining a sample.
- The patient must be instructed to collect a midstream sample. For certain tests, the first urine of the morning is preferred as it may have a higher concentrate of the component to be detected (e.g. Beta-hcg for pregnancy)
- If the patient is catheterized, the catheter usually has a sample port through which urine is collected.
- After proper hand decontamination and wearing gloves, the sample port is cleaned with an alcohol swab.
- The tube is clamped below the sample port to allow sufficient amount of urine to collect in the tube.
- A needle is then inserted in the sample port at 45 degrees, and aspirated to collect urine.
- The sample is then transferred immediately into a sterile container and sent to the laboratory.

OBTAINING A STOOL SAMPLE:

- Before obtaining the specimen, hands must first be decontaminated by thorough washing, and gloves and apron must be worn.

- The patient is asked to defecate into a clean bedpan or receiver.

- Requisite amount of stool (around 10 ml) is scooped up using the spoon provided, and transferred to the specimen container. The container lid must be closed immediately.

- The patient's hygiene must then be attended to, and gloves and waste must be discarded.

- Appropriate documentation, such as color and consistency of the stool, must be filled in prior to dispatching the specimen to the laboratory.

REFERENCES:

1. Dougherty, L., Lister, S. (2004) *The Royal Marsden Hospital Manual of Clinical Nursing Procedures* (6th ed). Oxford: Blackwell Publishing.

2. Colduvell, K. (2018). *How To Draw Blood Like A Pro: Step-By-Step Guide.* [online] Nurse.org. Available at: https://nurse.org/articles/how-nurses-professionally-draw-blood/ [Accessed 15 Jan. 2018].

EXERCISES:

1. What is the first step in obtaining a sample?
    a. Identifying the patient correctly
    b. Labeling the container
    c. Drawing blood
    d. Washing hands

2. Which blood test is generally done in newborn babies?
    a. Venous blood
    b. Finger stick
    c. Heel stick
    d. Arterial blood

3. How must the needle be inserted into the catheter to obtain a urine sample?
    a. Horizontally
    b. At 45 degrees
    c. At 90 degrees
    d. At 60 degrees

4. What is the proper amount of stool sample to be collected:
    a. 5 ml
    b. 10 ml

    c. 15 ml

    d. 20 ml

5. What types of samples can be analyzed in the laboratory?

    a. Blood

    b. Cerebrospinal fluid

    c. Synovial fluid

    d. All of the above

3. HEMATOLOGICAL TESTS

HEMOGRAM/COMPLETE BLOOD COUNT

The hemogram is a series of tests that provides information about all the components of the blood. This panel is used to evaluate a patient's overall health. It can detect a wide range of disorders from anemia and infections to rarer conditions. A list of the tests performed in a hemogram is outlined in Box 1. The details of individual tests are given below:

BOX 1. LIST OF TESTS PERFORMED IN A HEMOGRAM
Hemoglobin
Red blood cell count

Hematocrit/Packed cell volume

Red blood cell indices (MCV, MCH, MCHC)

Total white blood cell count

Differential count

Platelet count

TESTS FOR ANEMIA

Hemoglobin test:

- Hemoglobin is an iron containing protein that is found in red blood cells. It acts as a carrier for oxygen and carbon dioxide between the lungs and the various tissues of the body.
- Normal levels of hemoglobin are as follows:
    - Male: 12-17gms/100ml
    - Female: 11-15 gms/100ml
- Low hemoglobin is an indicator of anemia. It must be followed up with other tests for anemia (see Box 2).
- High hemoglobin levels are not very common but can occur, especially when oxygen levels are low, as can be seen in the following conditions:
    - At high altitudes
    - Diseases: Lung diseases like COPD, and smokers who may have pulmonary fibrosis.

- o It may also be seen in bone marrow diseases like polycythemia vera
- o Inappropriate use of certain drugs (e.g. Epoetin alfa)

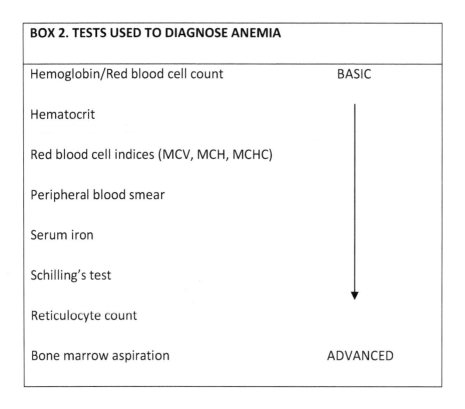

BOX 2. TESTS USED TO DIAGNOSE ANEMIA

Hemoglobin/Red blood cell count	BASIC
Hematocrit	
Red blood cell indices (MCV, MCH, MCHC)	
Peripheral blood smear	
Serum iron	
Schilling's test	
Reticulocyte count	
Bone marrow aspiration	ADVANCED

Red blood cell count:

- This count measures the amount of mature red blood cells present in the blood stream.
- Like hemoglobin, it can also serve as an indicator of anemia.
- Normal values:

- o Males: 4.5 to 6 million cells per cu mm of blood
- o Females: 4 to 5.5 million cells per cu mm of blood
- The causes for low and high blood values are similar to that of hemoglobin.

Packed cell volume (Hematocrit):

- The packed cell volume refers to the proportion of red blood cells that are present in a given sample of blood.
- The cells are 'packed' together by means of centrifugation and the resultant volume of cells is measured.
- Normal values:
  - o Males: 40-50%
  - o Females: 37-47%
- The hematocrit must always be taken in conjunction with the hemoglobin level, in order to interpret causes of increase or decrease in values.
- These are outlined in Box 3.

BOX 3. CAUSES OF CHANGE IN HEMATOCRIT LEVELS		
HEMATOCRIT	HEMOGLOBIN	CONDITIONS
Low	Low	Hemorrhage, anemia due to various causes

Low	Normal	Pregnancy, over-hydration
High	Normal	Dehydration
High	High	Low oxygen availability (high altitudes, smoking, pulmonary diseases) Polycythemia vera

Red blood cell indices (Wintrobe indices):

These indices are values that give specific information about the red blood cell such as its size and the concentration of hemoglobin within each cell. In the event of the above tests being abnormally low, the red blood indices can help to identify the specific cause of anemia. Following are the various red blood cell indices that are reported by laboratories:

- **Mean corpuscular volume (MCV):**
  - ○ This indicates the size or volume of a single red blood cell.
  - ○ The value is derived by dividing the patient's hematocrit (packed cell volume) by the red blood cell count.
  - ○ Normal value: 80-100 cubic microns
  - ○ This value helps to classify anemia based on the size of the RBC. For instance, a lower value will indicate small size of cells (Microcytic anemia), a normal

value may indicate a normocytic type, whereas a higher value will indicate large size of cells (Macrocytic anemia).

- **Mean corpuscular hemoglobin (MCH):**
  - This index indicates the amount or weight of hemoglobin present in a single red blood cell.
  - The value is derived by dividing the patient's hemoglobin level by the red blood cell count.
  - Normal value is 27-31 picograms/cell

- **Mean corpuscular hemoglobin concentration (MCHC):**

  - This index assesses both the size of the red blood cell as well as the concentration of hemoglobin within each cell.

  - This value is obtained by dividing the hemoglobin of the patient by the patient's hematocrit.

  - Normal value: 32-36 g/dl

  - Using this index, the anemia may be classified based on color (given by the hemoglobin present) as hypochromic, normochromic, or hyperchromic type.

BOX 4. SUMMARY OF NORMAL VALUES OF HEMATOLOGICAL TESTS DONE FOR ANEMIA.

	ADULT				CHILDREN	
	MALE		FEMALE			
	Normal range	Optimal Reading	Normal range	Optimal Reading	Normal range	Optimal Reading
HEMATOCRIT (HCT)	39-53%	46	36-49 %	41	51-61%	56
HEMOGLOBIN (HCB)	12-17 g/dl	14	13-16 g/dl	14	15-21 g/dl	17
Mean Corpuscular Hemoglobin (MCH)	27-33 pg.	30	27-33 pg.	30	Higher range in newborns and infants	
Mean Corpuscular Volume (MCV)	90-99 fl	90	90-99 fl	90	Higher range in newborns and infants	

Mean Corpuscular Hemoglobin Concentration (MCHC)	32-37 %	34	32-37 %	34	Higher range in newborns and infants
Red Blood Count (RBC)	4.2-5.6 mill/mc l	4.9	3.8-5.2 mill/mcl	4.55	Lower range in newborns and infants

ADVANCED TESTS FOR ANEMIA:

These are done to diagnose the specific etiology of anemia.

Peripheral blood smear:

- This gives information on the number, shape, and appearance of the red blood cells, which helps to identify the type of anemia, as given below:

BOX 5. INTERPRETING BLOOD SMEAR IN ANEMIA		
FEATURE	CHARACTERISTIC	TYPE OF ANEMIA
SIZE	Macrocytic	Megaloblastic anemia – folic acid and vitamin B12 deficiency
	Normocytic	Hemolytic anemia
	Microcytic	Iron deficiency, thalassemia, sideroblastic anemia
COLOR	Hypochromic (Target cell appearance)	Iron deficiency anemia
	Normochromic	Hemolytic anemia

- Shape of red blood cells is also studied. Normal cells have a biconcave disc appearance. This may be altered such as in spherocytosis, where red blood cells are of spherical shape.

Serum Iron:

- Iron forms an essential component of hemoglobin, and iron deficiency can therefore lead to anemia.
- Normal value: Males: 55 – 160 µg/dl

- Females: 40 - 155 µg/dl
- This value decreases in iron deficiency anemia.
- It may be increased in hemosiderosis, hemochromatosis, and certain anemias like hemolytic and pernicious anemia.

Schilling test:

- Absorption of vitamin B12 from the intestine requires the presence of a factor called intrinsic factor.
- If this is deficient, the body does not absorb vitamin B12, which would result in pernicious anemia.
- Radio labeled vitamin B12 is given orally. The patient's urine is then collected as a 24 hour sample and checked for levels of vitamin B12.
- In a normal patient, 8 to 40% of the radio labeled dose must be excreted, lesser amount is indicative of Pernicious anemia.

Reticulocyte count:

Reticulocytes are immature blood cells that normally account for 0.5% to 1.5% of the total RBC count.

It may increase if anemia is caused by destruction of red blood cells (hemolytic anemia).

Values are decreased in aplastic anemia and iron deficiency anemia.

Bone marrow aspiration:

- This is done only when the above tests are inconclusive.
- It is usually reserved for more serious forms of anemia.

NON SPECIFIC TESTS FOR INFECTION

White blood cells count:

- The white blood cells present in the blood stream serve as the body's defense mechanism against foreign bodies and infectious organisms.
- However, sometimes these cells may act against components of the hosts' body, thereby playing an important role in autoimmune diseases.
- Normal white cell count: 4500 – 10500 cells per cu mm of blood. However, it is usually higher in infants and children.
- The white blood cell count usually increases during infections. An extremely high rise in white blood cells can be an indication of malignant conditions such as leukemia.
- White blood cells are decreased during conditions of immunosuppression, due to various diseases or drugs.
- A white blood cell count is usually supported by a differential count, as detailed below.

Differential count:

There are five different types of white blood cells, each of which has a unique function.

The differential count gives the relative proportion of each of these white blood cells in the blood.

The proportion of various types of white blood cells, and the specific conditions in which they may be increased or decreased, are outlined in Box 6.

BOX 6. DIFFERENTIAL COUNT AND THEIR CLINICAL SIGNIFICANCE			
WHITE BLOOD CELL	PROPORTION	DECREASED IN	INCREASED IN
Neutrophils	40 – 75 %	Bone marrow depression due to radiation or chemotherapy Certain infections such as typhoid, measles, rubella systemic lupus erythematosus	Acute infections

Basophils	0 – 2 %	Hyperthyroidism Pregnancy and ovulation	Neoplasms like chronic myelocytic leukemia, polycythemia vera, Hodgkin's disease Chronic hypersensitivity conditions such as ulcerative colitis
Eosinophils	1 – 6 %	Stress due to trauma, surgery etc. Cushing's syndrome	Allergies Parasitic infections Skin diseases Some neoplasms, e.g. Hodgkin's disease, myelocytic leukemia

Lymphocytes	20 – 25 %	Congestive cardiac failure, renal failure, corticosteroid therapy	Infections such as tuberculosis, syphilis and pertussis Autoimmune diseases and ulcerative colitis
Monocytes	2 – 10 %	---	Infections such as bacterial endocarditis, tuberculosis, etc. Autoimmune diseases such as rheumatoid arthritis and systemic lupus erythematosus.

TESTS FOR BLOOD COAGULATION:

Coagulation tests are used to find out how fast the blood clots. There are both non-specific and specific tests for coagulation. Non-specific tests are usually done only for general screening, as a part of routine medical check-up or prior to surgery. Specific tests are used only when the results of non-specific tests are abnormal, or if specific indications exist.

The non-specific tests for blood coagulation are as follows:

Bleeding time:

- This basically tests how long it takes a patient to stop bleeding. This test is an indicator of how well the platelets are functioning.
- Bleeding is induced in the patient by lacerating the forearm (Ivy method) or placing a small prick on the earlobe or finger (Duke method). The blood is blotted with a filter paper every 30 seconds and time taken to stop bleeding is measured.
- Normal values:
  - Ivy method: 1 to 6 minutes
  - Duke method: 1 to 3 minutes

Clotting time:

- This test measures the time taken for the blood to coagulate outside the body (in vitro), under standard conditions.
- Blood is usually collected and placed in a capillary tube or test tube. The time taken for it to clot is assessed.
- Normal value: 8 to 15 minutes.

If the bleeding time and clotting time have been found to be abnormal, the cause of abnormal coagulation must be ascertained. In these cases, a series of specific tests is done. In order to decide which test is to be used, knowledge of the normal mechanism of coagulation is essential. This is outlined in Figure 1.

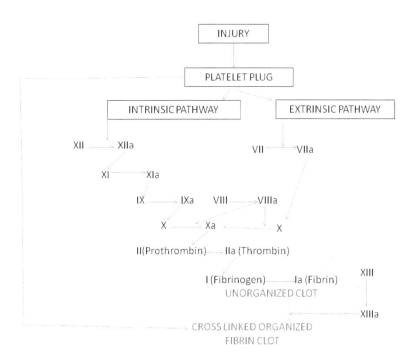

Figure 1. Normal clotting mechanism

Based on each step of the above flowchart, specific tests for coagulation may be carried out. Specific tests are also indicated when patient has unexplained bruising or has clinically observed prolonged bleeding. They may also be used to test the effectiveness of anticoagulant therapies.

These tests are outlined below:

Platelet count:

- Platelets are the third group of cells found in whole blood and they play an important role in initial clotting of blood after injury.
- Platelet count measures the actual number of platelets present in the blood. It does not, however, give a clear picture of platelet function.
- Normal platelet count: 150,000 to 350,000 per cu mm of blood
- Platelet count can be decreased as a result of certain viral infections (e.g. Dengue)and drugs (antineoplastic drugs). It can increase during cold weather, at high altitudes, and after strenuous exercise.

Partial thromboplastin time (PTT) and activated partial thromboplastin time (aPTT):

- Both the above tests are essentially the same. In aPTT, an activator is added to the blood sample to speed up the clotting time. Therefore, the reference range is narrower.
- The aPTT tests the efficacy of both the intrinsic and common pathway. This test evaluates Factors I, II, V, VIII, IX, X, XI and XII.
- Normal values:

- o aPTT: 30 – 40 seconds
- o PTT: 60 – 70 seconds
- This test may be prolonged in the following conditions:
    - o Hereditary diseases like hemophilia A and B, and von Willebrand disease
    - o Vitamin K deficiency (which aids in synthesis of certain clotting factors)
    - o Liver cirrhosis (most clotting factors are synthesized in the liver)
    - o Anticoagulant drug therapy
    - o If the aPTT is shortened, it may be indicative of disseminated intravascular coagulation. It also decreases after severe hemorrhage and in extensive cancer.

Prothrombin time and International Normalized Ratio (INR):

- Prothrombin time measures the efficacy of the extrinsic pathway and the common pathway.
- It tests factors II, VII, V and X.
- The prothrombin time has significant interlaboratory variability due to differences in the reagent used (usually calcium and thromboplastin). In order to offset this and establish standardization, the INR was introduced.
- Normal prothrombin time: 9.5 seconds to 13.5 seconds.

- The mean prothrombin time for a specific population is calculated by using the sensitivity index given by the manufacturer. The INR is then determined by dividing the patient's prothrombin time with the mean prothrombin time. Ideally, the patient's INR must be equal to 1. However, a reference value up to 1.3 is usually considered normal.

- Prothrombin time may be increased in the following conditions:
  - Use of anticoagulant drugs
  - Liver diseases
  - Vitamin K deficiency
  - Disseminated intravascular coagulation
  - Massive blood transfusions
  - Hypothermia

- It may be decreased during transfusion of fresh frozen plasma or on vitamin K supplementation.

Plasma fibrinogen:

- This test measures the levels of fibrinogen present in the blood. It is usually done when the results of both PT/INR and aPTT are abnormal. It is also used when abnormal thrombotic events are suspected (e.g. DIC).

- Normal levels: 150 – 400 mg/dl

- The levels may be decreased in end-stage liver disease, afibrinogenemia, hypofibrinogenemia, DIC, and large blood transfusion.
- It may be increased in inflammatory conditions, trauma or cancers.

D-Dimer tests:

- Unlike the above tests, which are done to detect causes of increased bleeding, the D-dimer test is done to detect abnormal coagulation of blood.
- It is indicated in patients who are suspected of having thrombotic events (e.g., those who are suspected of having deep vein thrombosis and/or pulmonary embolism), and those who have signs of disseminated intravascular coagulation.
- D-dimers are formed in the blood as an end product of degradation of the fibrin clot, and would be present only if the coagulation pathway has been activated.
- A D-dimer value that is less than 500 ng/ml excludes the possibility of the patient having venous thromboembolism (DVT or PE). However, if the D-dimer value is above this level, additional tests to detect DVT and PE must be performed, such as ultrasound or lung CT scans.

BLOOD GROUPING AND TYPING:

ABO grouping:

- This is done to determine an individual's blood type.

- Depending on the types of antigens present on the red blood cells, the blood groups are classified as A, B, AB, and O type.

- The type of antigens expressed on RBCs and blood type is determined genetically. A and B type antigens are expressed from dominant genes and O from recessive genes.

- Individuals tend to produce antibodies against antigens that are not expressed on their red blood cells. So if cells containing those antigens enter the bloodstream accidentally, (e.g. during transfusion of another blood type), they are destroyed by these antibodies.

- Therefore, ABO testing must be performed prior to any blood transfusion to avoid severe transfusion reactions.

A list of genotype, phenotype, and antibodies is described in Box 7.

BOX 7. PROPERTIES OF BLOOD GROUP ANTIGENS

BLOOD GROUP/ PHENOTYPE	GENOTYPE	ANTIGENS ON RBCs	ANTIBODIES PRODUCED
A	AA, AO	A Antigen	Anti-B
B	BB, BO	B antigen	Anti-A
AB	AB	Both A and B antigen	None
O	OO	None	Anti-A and Anti-B

Rh typing:

- Rhesus protein is another antigen that can be present on red blood cells.
- If the cells have the Rh antigen, an individual is said to be Rh positive, and if the individual lacks this antigen, the individual is said to be Rh negative.
- Similar to ABO groups, an Rh negative individual can produce antibodies (anti-Rh) to the Rh antigen.
- This is clinically significant when an Rh negative mother has an Rh positive fetus for the second time.

- The mother can produce antibodies to the Rh antigen of the first baby, when the blood gets exposed to the Rh antigen during delivery.

- These antibodies might cross the placenta during the second pregnancy and damage the RBCs of the second fetus.

- This disease is referred to as hemolytic disease of the newborn, and needs to be avoided by prior sensitization to the antigen.

REFERENCES:

1. Normal Ranges for Common Laboratory Tests. Available at http://rml.rush.edu/Pages/RMLRanges.aspx.

2. Laboratory reference range values. Available at http://www.stedmansonline.com/webFiles/Dict-Stedmans28/APP17.pdf.

3. Farinde, A. (2018). *Lab Values, Normal Adult: Laboratory Reference Ranges in Healthy Adults*. [online] Emedicine.medscape.com. Available at: https://emedicine.medscape.com/article/2172316-overview [Accessed 15 Jan. 2018].

4. Hematological and immunological tests. (1979). *Burns*, *5*(3), 286. http://dx.doi.org/10.1016/0305-4179(79)90089-5

5. Moll, R., & Davis, B. (2017). Iron, vitamin B 12 and folate. *Medicine*.

6. Dean L., M.D. Blood Group and Red Cell Antigens. NCBI. Available at http://www.ncbi.nlm.nih.gov.bookshelf/br.fcgi?=bookrbc antigen&part=ch05ABO. Accessed: January 2018.

EXERCISES:

1. Which of the following would indicate anemia?
   a. Male has RBC 3.2 million/mcL
   b. Female has RBC 3.2 million/mcL
   c. Male has 5.8 million/mcl RBC cells
   d. Female has 5.8 million cells/mcL RBC

2. Cause of iron-deficiency anemia would be:
   a. Not drinking milk daily
   b. Does not include leafy vegetables or meat
   c. Does not do exercises
   d. Does not drink enough water with the food

3. How many platelets should be there in a unit of blood?
   a. 5,000 – 10,000
   b. 50,000 – 200,000
   c. 150,000 – 450,000
   d. 200,000 – 300,000

4. What is the normal lab value for lymphocytes?
   a. 500 – 600
   b. 1000 – 4000
   c. 2000 – 5000
   d. 10,000 – 200,000

5. A nurse is reviewing the complete blood count (CBC) of a child who has been diagnosed with idiopathic thrombocytopenic purpura. Which of the following laboratory result should the nurse report immediately to the physician?

    a. Platelet count of 30,000/mm3.

    b. Hemoglobin level of 7.5 g/dL.

    c. Reticulocyte count of 6.5%.

    d. Eosinophil count of 700 cells/mm3.

6. An adult male with hemoglobin count of 12.5 g/dL most likely has which of the following conditions?

    a. Emphysema.

    b. Client living at a high altitude.

    c. Dehydration.

    d. History of an enlarged spleen.

7. Which of the following indices measures the concentration of hemoglobin in the red blood cells?

    a. MCV

    b. MCH

    c. MCHC

    d. ESR

8. What does the hematocrit measure?

    a. Measures WBC in total blood volume

    b. Measures RBC in total blood volume

    c. Measures platelets in total blood volume

    d. Measures Hb in total blood volume

9. Which of the following conditions does cause a rise in neutrophil levels?

    a. Parasitic infections

    b. Acute infections

    c. Autoimmune diseases

    d. Allergies

10. Partial thromboplastin time measures which component of the coagulation pathway?

    a. Platelet aggregation

    b. Intrinsic pathway

    c. Extrinsic pathway

    d. Fibrinolytic pathway

11. Which of the following blood groups can be transfused to an AB
    blood type

        a. A

        b. B

        c. O

        d. All of the above

4. TESTS FOR ENDOCRINE FUNCTION

TESTS FOR DIABETES

Diabetes mellitus is one of the most common diseases in the developed world, caused due to ineffective secretion of the insulin hormone from the pancreas, which is responsible for metabolism of glucose. Early and effective detection and management is crucial as sustained high blood glucose levels can cause damage to various body organs such as the kidneys, nerves, eyes, and blood vessels. Laboratory tests for diabetes may be indicated in the following situations:

- When the patient presents with suspicious signs of diabetes such as increased appetite, increased thirst, or increased frequency of urination (polyphagia, polydipsia, and polyuria).

- To monitor a known diabetic to ensure that treatment is effective.
- In the emergency room if extremes of blood sugar levels are suspected.

A list of laboratory tests performed are given below:

Random blood sugar (RBS):

- This test can be taken at any time of the day, regardless of when the patient has last eaten. The results, however, may not be sensitive as it would depend on the patient's food intake.
- It is generally used as a screening test or in emergency situations.
- A random blood sugar level that is greater than 11.1 mmol/l or 200mg/dl is suggestive of diabetes.

Fasting blood sugar (FBS):

- This test must be performed when the patient is fasting, that is, the patient should not have consumed anything (except water) for eight hours prior to giving the test sample.
- The results of the test must be interpreted as follows:

- o Normal: 70 – 99 mg/dl or 3.9 – 5.5 mmol/l
- o Pre-diabetes: 100 – 125 mg/dl or 5.6 – 6.5 mmol/l
- o Diabetes: Greater than 126 mg/dl or 7 mmol/l on more than one test sample

Postprandial blood sugar (PPS):

- This test is done two hours after the patient has eaten a meal.
- When the patient eats, the blood glucose increases slightly, which stimulate the pancreas to release insulin. This in turn metabolizes the glucose and clears it from the blood within two hours. Therefore the postprandial blood sugar test is useful in assessing insulin function. Patients who have insulin resistance may have normal fasting levels but increased postprandial levels of blood glucose.
- A postprandial blood sugar range of more than 140 mg/dl is indicative of impaired insulin function, and whether the patients' drug dosage regimen is appropriate.

Oral glucose tolerance test:

- This test must also be done under fasting conditions. It tests the body's ability to tolerate glucose load. It may be a single step or two step test.
- After the fasting blood sample is taken, the patient consumes a glucose drink. Blood samples are then repeated after one

hour (for two-step test) and then after two hours. In a single step test, the sample is taken only after two hours.

- This test is especially useful for diagnosing pre-diabetes, and screening pregnant women for gestational diabetes.
- As with the postprandial blood tests, the results after two hours can be interpreted as follows:
  - o Normal: Less than 140 mg/dl (7.8 mmol/l)
  - o Pre-diabetes or impaired glucose tolerance: 140 – 200 mg/dl (7.8 – 11 mmol/l)
  - o Diabetes: Greater than 200 mg/dl (11.1 mmol/l)

Glycosylated hemoglobin test (HbA1c):

- This test works on the principle that a certain amount of glucose is always attached to the hemoglobin within red blood cells. This amount depends on the amount of glucose present in the bloodstream, and would increase in diabetics.
- Since the lifespan of an RBC is 120 days, this test value would reflect the patient's glycemic control over the past three months.
- The test value can be interpreted as follows:
  - o Normal: Less than 5.7%
  - o Prediabetes: 5.7% to 6.4%
  - o Diabetes: greater than 6.5%
- This test is also commonly used to monitor blood glucose status of known diabetic patients, so that the efficacy of their

drug regimen may be assessed and changed if required. The recommended goal for diabetic is below 7%.

TESTS FOR THYROID AND PARATHYROID FUNCTION

Thyroid function tests:

- The thyroid hormone plays an important role in regulating metabolic processes within the body. Increase or decrease of these hormones can affect the body's normal metabolic rate.

- If an increase or decrease of these hormones is suspected clinically, thyroid function tests may be performed.

- Decrease in thyroid hormone levels slows the body metabolism and is referred to as hypothyroidism. This may be manifested by weight gain, depression, or lack of energy.

- Increase in thyroid hormone levels is associated with increased metabolism that might be manifested as weight loss, anxiety, tremors, and nervousness.

- There are two hormones secreted by the thyroid gland – T3 (Triiodothyronine) and T4 (Thyroxine). The levels of these hormones are measured in the blood. Apart from this, the thyroid stimulating hormone (TSH) is a hormone released by the pituitary gland. It stimulates the thyroid gland to release T3 and T4, and functions by a negative feedback mechanism. Therefore, its levels would be high if T3 and T4 levels are low, and vice-versa.

- The normal values for various thyroid hormones and conditions in which variations are seen have been summarized in Box 1.

BOX 1. SUMMARY OF THYROID HORMONE LEVELS				
THYROID HORMONE	NORMAL RANGE	OPTIMAL READING	DECREASED LEVELS	INCREASED LEVELS
THYROXINE (T4)	4 – 12 ug/dl	8 ug/dl	Chronic thyroiditis, malnutrition, cirrhosis, hypothyroidism, cretinism	Hepatitis, acute thyroiditis, hyperthyroidi-sm
T3 -UPTAKE	27 – 47 %	37%	Pregnancy, hyperestrogeni-sm, hypothyroidism.	Severe liver disease, pulmonary insufficiency, hyperthyroidi-sm, metastatic malignancies
THYROID-STIMULATI	0.5 – 6	-	Raised T3, T4	Lowered T3, T4

NG HORMONE (TSH)	mill U/L		levels	levels.
FREE T4 INDEX (T7)	4 -12	8		

TESTS FOR PARATHYROID FUNCTION:

Serum parathyroid hormone (PTH):

- This hormone plays an important role in calcium metabolism in the body. It is released in response to low serum metabolism. Its functions are:
  - Signaling the bones to release calcium into the bloodstream
  - Signaling the kidneys to reabsorb calcium into the body and excrete phosphorous.
  - It also helps in activation of vitamin D
- Normal values: 10 – 65 ng/L
- Hyperparathyroidism causes increased PTH, which usually occurs in tumors of the parathyroid.
- Hypoparathyroidism can occur after surgical removal of the glands.

TESTS FOR ADRENAL FUNCTION:

The adrenal gland is composed of the cortex, which releases mineralocorticoid (aldosterone), and the medulla, which releases glucocorticoids (cortisol). These are released after stimulation by the adrenocorticotropic hormone released by the anterior pituitary. In cases of adrenal malfunction, the following laboratory tests are performed:

ACTH test:

- Normal ACTH levels are as follows:
    - Males: 7 – 50 pg/ml
    - Females: 5 – 27 pg/ml
- Decreased levels indicate a pituitary deficit.

Adrenal stimulation test:

- The adrenal gland is stimulated by injecting synthetic ACTH or cosyntropin.
- The amount of cortisol and aldosterone produced is measured.
- Baseline value for cortisol is 20 – 30 μg/dl, and is 20 ng/dl for aldosterone. If the cortisol fails to double from the baseline, it is indicative of adrenal insufficiency.

Normal levels of other important hormones:

The laboratory values of other important hormones are detailed below:

BOX 2. LABORATORY VALUES OF IMPORTANT HORMONES	
HORMONE	NORMAL RANGE
Growth hormone	0 – 5 ng/ml
Follicle stimulating hormone	Male: 1 – 10 IU/l Female: Follicular/Luteal phase: 1 – 10 IU/l Ovulation: 5 – 25 IU/l Post-menopausal: 30 – 110 IU/l
Prolactin	< 14 ng/ml
Progesterone	70 – 280 ng/dl
Estradiol	Male: 1.5 – 5 ng/dl Female: Follicular phase: 2 -14 ng/dl Luteal phase: 2 – 16 ng/dl Post-menopausal: < 3.5 ng/dl
Testosterone	10 – 25 nmol/l

REFERENCES:

1) Sacks, D. B., Bruns, D. E., Goldstein, D. E., Maclaren, N. K., McDonald, J. M., & Parrott, M. (2002). Guidelines and recommendations for laboratory analysis in the diagnosis and management of diabetes mellitus. *Clinical chemistry*, *48*(3), 436-472.

2) Surks, M. I., Chopra, I. J., Mariash, C. N., Nicoloff, J. T., & Solomon, D. H. (1990). American Thyroid Association guidelines for use of laboratory tests in thyroid disorders. *Jama*, *263*(11), 1529-1532.

3) Poole KE, Reeve J. Parathyroid hormone - a bone anabolic and catabolic agent. *Curr Opin Pharmacol*. 2005 Dec. 5(6):612-7. [Medline].

4) Fischbach FT, Dunning MB III, eds. *Manual of Laboratory and Diagnostic Tests*. 8th ed. Philadelphia: Lippincott Williams and Wilkins.: 2009.

5) Simsek Y, Karaca Z, Tanriverdi F, Unluhizarci K, Selcuklu A, Kelestimur F. A comparison of low-dose ACTH, glucagon stimulation and insulin tolerance test in patients with pituitary disorders. *Clin Endocrinol (Oxf)*. 2014 Jun 20

EXERCISES:

1. Which of the following represents normal fasting blood sugar range?

    a. 120 – 140 mg/dl

    b. 140 – 160 mg/dl

    c. 50 – 70 mg/dl

    d. 70 – 100 mg/dl

2. Which test is the best for long-term monitoring of diabetic patients?

    a. Fasting blood sugar

    b. Glycosylated hemoglobin

    c. Random blood sugar

    d. Oral glucose tolerance test

3. Which of the following is not a test that is used for the diagnosis of diabetes?

    a. Oral glucose tolerance test

    b. Glycosylated hemoglobin

    c. Insulin tolerance test

    d. Fasting blood glucose

4. Which of the following values is an abnormal value of thyroxine hormone?

    a. 4 µg/dl

    b. 6 µg/dl

    c. 12 µg/dl

    d. 15 µg/dl

5. Which of the following is not a function of the parathyroid hormone?

    a. Activation of vitamin D

    b. Release of calcium from bones

    c. Excretion of phosphorous by kidney

    d. Increasing the basal metabolic rate

5. TESTS FOR LIVER AND GASTROINTESTINAL FUNCTION

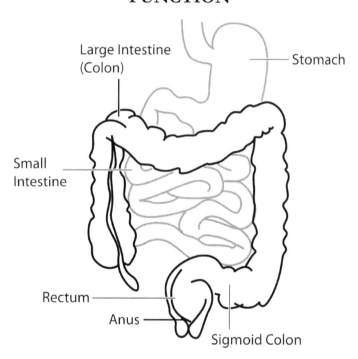

This is a series of tests that is done to assess how well the liver is functioning. It measures certain proteins and enzymes that are normally released by liver cells.

These tests are usually performed in patients who are known to have or are suspected of having liver disease, including:

- Patients with clinical signs of jaundice

- Chronic alcoholics

- Patients with viral infections like hepatitis, particularly hepatitis B.

The various components tested are outlined below:

Serum bilirubin:

- Bilirubin is a breakdown product of hemoglobin. Its unconjugated form passes to the liver, where it is conjugated and subsequently excreted largely through the urine.
- Both the conjugated (direct) form and unconjugated (indirect) form can be measured from serum.
- Normal value:
    - Total bilirubin: 0.2 – 1.2 mg/dl
    - Direct bilirubin: 0.1 – 0.4 mg/dl

o   Indirect bilirubin: 0.4– 1.1 mg/dl

Elevated bilirubin level is indicative of jaundice, which could be due to several reasons (See Box 1).

BOX 1. CAUSES OF ELEVATED BILIRUBIN			
TYPE OF BILIRUBIN ELEVATED	TYPE OF JAUNDICE PRESENT	OTHER FINDINGS	CAUSES
Unconjugated bilirubin	Pre – hepatic	Increased urobilinogen in urine	Increased hemolysis – newborns, malaria, sickle cell anemia, thalessemia, hemolytic – uremic syndrome
Both conjugated and unconjugated bilirubin	Hepatic	Dark urine (due to urobilinogen and conjugated bilirubin), slightly pale stools	Hepatitis, cirrhosis, alcoholic liver disease

Conjugated bilirubin	Post – hepatic	Dark urine, pale stools	Gallstones, bile duct strictures, biliary atresia, pancreatic cancer

Serum Albumin:

- Albumin is a plasma protein that maintains the oncotic pressure of the blood and also aids in transport of a variety of proteins and hormones.
- Normal value: 3.5 – 5.5 g/dl.
- Serum albumin levels may be decreased in the following conditions:
  - Liver diseases – hepatitis, cirrhosis, ascites
  - Kidney diseases – glomerulonephritis, nephropathy
  - Malnutrition, malabsorption syndromes
  - Burn injuries
- Higher levels of albumin are usually associated with dehydration.

Serum globulin:

- Globulin is another serum protein that is of three types – alpha, beta, and gamma. These proteins have a wide variety of functions, including hemoglobin binding, transport, and immune functions.

- Normal values:
  - o Alpha-1 globulin: 0.1 – 0.3 g/dl
  - o Alpha-2 globulin: 0.6 – 1.0 g/dl
  - o Beta globulin: 0.7 – 1.1 g/dl

Albumin/Globulin ratio:

- Usually albumin makes up 60% of the blood's protein while globulin makes up around 40%.
- The normal A/G ratio is 0.8 to 2.0.
- If, however, either the albumin is lowered, or globulins increase for various reasons, this ratio can be altered.
- This would be seen in chronic inflammatory diseases, multiple myeloma, and autoimmune diseases such as rheumatoid arthritis.

A summary of the various serum proteins is outlined below:

BOX 2. SERUM PROTEIN LEVELS		
	NORMAL RANGE	**OPTIMAL READING**
PROTEIN TOTAL	6 – 8.5 g/dl	7.25

ALBUMIN	3.2 – 5.0 g/dl	4.1
GLOBULIN	2.2 – 4.2 g/dl (calculated)	3.2
ALBUMIN/GLOBULIN RATIO (A/G RATIO)	0.8 – 2.0 (calculated)	1.9

Alkaline Phosphatase:

- Alkaline phosphatase is an enzyme that is present not only in the liver, but also in the bone and intestine. This enzyme had many metabolic functions, and is believed to play an important role in skeletal mineralization.
- Normal values: 20-140 IU/L
- Increased levels of alkaline phosphatase may be found in the following conditions:
  - Liver diseases – Cirrhosis, hepatitis, biliary obstruction
  - Bone diseases – Bone tumors, osteoporosis, rickets, Paget's disease and hyperparathyroidism
  - Other malignancies like leukemias and lymphomas
- Decreased levels of alkaline phosphatase may be seen in:
  - Diseases like Wilson's disease, hyperphosphatasia, cretinism etc.

- Blood disorders like pernicious anemia, aplastic anemia and chronic myelogenous leukemia

.

Aspartate aminotransferase:

- This is also known as Serum glutamic oxaloacetic transaminase (SGOT)
- This enzyme is largely present in the liver and heart, but may also be seen in the kidney, brain, muscles, and red blood cells. If any of these structures is damaged, it could be reflected by an increase in this enzyme.
- Decreased values of AST may be seen in congested liver, or in patients with high cholesterol levels.
- Increased values may be due to various causes as follows:
  - Liver diseases, alcoholism,
  - Myocardial infarction
  - Kidney infections and diseases
- A rise in the level of AST must always be taken in conjunction with ALT levels. If ALT is normal, then, rather than liver disease, it indicates damage to some other organ, for example, cardiac muscle.

Alanine transaminase:

- This enzyme is also known as Serum glutamic pyruvate transaminase (SGPT).
- Unlike AST, this enzyme is more specific for liver function. It is found primarily in the liver and kidney.
- Normal value: 20 – 60 IU/L
- It is elevated in liver diseases. The AST:ALT ratio can be used to detect alcohol-induced liver disease. An AST:ALT value of greater than 2 is indicative of this condition. This is called De Ritis ratio.

Gamma glutaryl transferase:

- This enzyme is found in the liver, kidney, and pancreas. Although it is present in higher amounts in the kidney, its activity is greater in the liver.
- Normal value: 0 – 30 IU/L
- Increased levels of GGT are usually associated with the following conditions:
  - Liver diseases – cirrhosis, hepatitis, alcoholic liver disease, liver cancer
  - Cancers of the prostate, breast, and lung
  - Pancreatitis
  - Systemic lupus erythematosus

- The GGT levels may be used along with elevated alkaline phosphatase levels to determine the disease source. If both GGT and ALP are elevated, it is indicative of hepatobiliary disease, whereas, an isolated increase in ALP suggests bone disease.

- GGT levels may be decreased in hyperthyroidism, hypothalamic dysfunction, or low magnesium levels.

A summary of the various hepatic enzymes and their normal levels is given in Box 3.

BOX 3. HEPATIC ENZYMES – NORMAL LEVELS				
HEPATIC ENZYMES	**ADULT**		**CHILDREN**	
	NORMAL RANGE	**OPTIMAL READING**	**NORMAL RANGE**	**OPTIMAL READING**
AST (serum glutamic-oxaloacetic transaminase - SGOT)	0 – 42 U/L	21	-	-

ALT (serum glutamic-pyruvic transaminase - SGPT)	0 – 48 U/L		24		-	-
Alkaline phosphatase	20 – 125 U/L		72.5		40–400 U/L	220
GGT (gamma-glutamyl transpeptidase)	0 – 45 U/L	22.5	0 – 65 U/L	32.5	-	-
LDH (lactic acid dehydrogenase)	0 – 250 U/L		125		-	-
BILIRUBIN, TOTAL	0 – 1.3 mg/dl		0.65		-	-

REFERENCES:

1. Westwood, A. The analysis of bilirubin in serum. *Annals of clinical biochemistry*. 1991. 28(2):119.

2. Chopra, S., & Griffin, P. H. (1985). Laboratory tests and diagnostic procedures in evaluation of liver disease. *The American journal of medicine, 79*(2), 221-230.

3. Lum G, Gambino SR. Serum gamma-glutamyl transpeptidase activity as an indicator of disease of liver, pancreas, or bone. *Clin Chem.* 1972 Apr. 18(4):358-62.

4. Sharma U, Pal D, Prasad R. Alkaline phosphatase: an overview. Ind J clin Biochem 2014; 29 (3) : 269 – 278

5. Cohen, J. A., & Kaplan, M. M. (1979). The SGOT/SGPT ratio—an indicator of alcoholic liver disease. *Digestive diseases and sciences, 24*(11), 835-838.

6. Hoofnagle JH, Van Natta ML, Kleiner DE, Clark JM, Kowdley KV, Loomba R, et al. Vitamin E and changes in serum alanine aminotransferase levels in patients with non-alcoholic steatohepatitis. *Aliment Pharmacol Ther.* 2013 Jul. 38(2):134-43

EXERCISES:

1. Which of the following is not a normal value of Gamma Glutamyl transferase?

   a. 5 U/l

   b. 25 U/l

   c. 55 U/l

   d. 75 U/l

2. The De Ritis ratio, used to detect alcoholic liver disease, is the ratio between which of the following?

   a. AST: ALT

   b. ALP: ACP

   c. Albumin: Globulin

   d. Conjugated bilirubin: Unconjugated Bilirubin

3. Conjugated bilirubin does not rise in which of the following conditions?

   a. Hepatitis

   b. Sickle cell anemia

   c. Gallstones

   d. Pancreatic cancer

4. Which of the following is the correct range for albumin: globulin ratio?

   a. 0.2 – 0.5

b. $0.8 - 2.0$

c. $6.0 - 8.0$

d. $2.0 - 3.5$

5. A rise in levels of Serum Glutamic Oxaloacetic aminotransferase (SGOT) is seen in all the following conditions except:

a. Paget's disease

b. Renal failure

c. Myocardial infarction

d. Cirrhosis

6. TESTS FOR RENAL FUNCTION

Blood urea nitrogen:

- In the body, unutilized proteins and amino acids are generally broken down by the liver into urea and carbon dioxide. T

- The urea is usually excreted by renal tubules. If the kidney fails to function, the levels of urea in the blood can increase. BUN is inversely proportional to the glomcrular filtration rate.

- Therefore, blood urea nitrogen (BUN) levels are a reflection of liver and renal function.

- Normal values of BUN: 3 – 20 mg/dl

- Increased levels of BUN occur due to kidney damage, low fluid intake, exercise, high protein intake, certain drugs, heart failure, or intestinal bleeding.
- Low levels are seen when the person has a low nitrogen diet, liver damage, malabsorption, or poor diet.

Serum Creatinine:

- Creatinine is a dehydration product of creatine present in the muscle, and is formed at a constant rate.
- It is freely filtered by the glomerulus and does not get either reabsorbed or secreted again.
- Therefore, it is an efficient measure of the kidney's glomerular filtration rate.
- Normal values:
    - Males: 0.5 – 1.2 mg/dl
    - Females: 0.4 – 1.1 mg/dl
    - Children: 0.0 – 0.7 mg/dl
- Its values are increased when the GFR decreases, as in acute or chronic kidney disease. Certain drugs that block kidney function might induce high levels of creatinine. This also happens when the person has muscle degeneration.
- Its values are decreased when the muscle mass is low. We also see low levels when a woman is pregnant, a person has protein starvation, or liver disease.

- 24 hour creatinine clearance is also measured along with this test. Urine sample is collected for 24 hours and the amount of creatinine excreted in this sample is determined.
- Normal range: 500 – 2000 mg/day

Uric acid:

- Uric acid is the final breakdown product of purine catabolism. It is produced by the liver and two thirds is eliminated by the kidney, with the rest being eliminated by the gastrointestinal tract.
- Normal values:
  - Males: 2.5 – 8 mg/dl
  - Females: 1.9 – 7.5 mg/dl
- Although it can be raised in renal failure, it is not a useful marker as it is also increased in other numerous conditions such as gout, metabolic and lactic acidosis, parathyroid disease etc.

BUN: Creatinine ratio:

This ratio is used to determine the cause of kidney disease.

While both BUN and creatinine are freely filtered by the glomerulus, urea alone is reabsorbed, whereas creatinine is not. This helps us determine the cause of kidney injury.

This is outlined in Box 1 below

BOX 1: BUN:CREATININE RATION TO DETERMINE CAUSE OF RENAL DISEASE		
LOCATION OF DISEASE	PROBLEM	BUN:CREATININE RATIO
Pre-renal	Dehydration, hypoperfusion	> 20:1
Post-renal	Obstructive diseases such as renal calculi, strictures	10 – 20:1
Renal	Renal damage	< 10:1

REFERENCES:

1. Prigent, A. (2008, January). Monitoring renal function and limitations of renal function tests. In *Seminars in nuclear medicine* (Vol. 38, No. 1, pp. 32-46). WB Saunders.

2. Gowda, S., Desai, P. B., Kulkarni, S. S., Hull, V. V., Math, A. A., & Vernekar, S. N. (2010). Markers of renal function tests. *North American journal of medical sciences*, *2*(4), 170.

3. Dossetor, J. B. (1966). Creatininemia versus uremia: the relative significance of blood urea nitrogen and serum creatinine concentrations in azotemia. *Annals of Internal Medicine*, *65*(6), 1287-1299.

4. Finco, D. R., & Duncan, J. R. (1976). Evaluation of blood urea nitrogen and serum creatinine concentrations as indicators of renal dysfunction: a study of 111 cases and a review of related literature. *Journal of the American Veterinary Medical Association*, *168*(7), 593-601.

EXERCISES:

1. Which of the following tests is not an efficient marker for renal function?
   a. Blood urea nitrogen
   b. Creatinine
   c. BUN: Creatinine ratio
   d. Uric acid

2. Which of the following is a post-renal cause for kidney failure?
   a. Nephrotoxic drugs
   b. Renal calculi
   c. Glomerulonephritis
   d. All of the above

3. Uric acid is produced as a breakdown product of which of the following compounds?
   a. Purines
   b. Pyramidines
   c. Proteins
   d. Carbohydrates

4. Which of the following values is not considered normal in a 24 hour creatinine clearance test?
   a. 500 mg per day

    b. 1500 mg per day

    c. 2000 mg per day

    d. 3500 mg per day

5. Which is the normal reference range for Blood Urea Nitrogen?

    a. 13 – 40 mg/dl

    b. 3 – 20 mg/dl

    c. 23 – 60 mg/dl

    d. 53 – 90 mg/dl

7. TESTS FOR SERUM ELECTROLYTES

Electrolytes refer to various ions in the body that are responsible for regulation of several functions, including proper muscle and nerve function. Electrolytes exist as both cations and anions, and, in order to maintain homeostasis, the values of these ions must be balanced with each other in the blood as well as with those present in the intracellular fluid. There are several electrolytes in the body. The important ones have been described below:

Sodium:

- Sodium alone accounts for 95% of the electrolytes present in the extracellular fluid. It plays an important role in regulating osmotic and acid-base balance of the body.

- Regulation of sodium levels is done primarily by the kidney using hormones like aldosterone and atrial natriuretic peptide (ANP).
- Normal value: 135 – 145 mmol/l
- Increased sodium (hypernatremia) can occur when:
  - Decreased body water – impaired thirst mechanism, diabetes insipidus
  - Increased mineralocorticoids – Cushing's disease, hyperaldosteronism etc.
- Decreased sodium (hyponatremia) can occur when:
  - Increased body fluids – heart failure, ascites etc
  - Decreased mineralocorticoid secretion – adrenal insufficiency

Potassium:

- As potassium is primarily an intracellular electrolyte, its levels in plasma tend to be low
- Normal value:3.5 – 5 meQ/l
- It is critical to normal nerve and muscle function (including cardiac muscle), and therefore it has a very narrow reference range.
- If potassium values move outside of these levels, arrhythmias or irregular heartbeat can result; therefore potassium levels must be monitored very closely.

- Potassium is also affected by the hormone aldosterone. It is inversely related to sodium levels. If sodium levels decrease, potassium levels tend to increase, and vice-versa.
- The cause of increased potassium levels (hyperkalemia) is not clear.
- Decreased potassium levels (hypokalemia) can occur in dehydration, vomiting, and acetaminophen overdose.

Calcium:

- Calcium is an important element of the human body, and makes up approximately 2% of body weight.
- Calcium has several functions, which include the following:
- Mineralization of bones in the body
- Aiding in blood coagulation
- Playing a role in heart and skeletal muscle contractility.
- Normal laboratory values for calcium are:
- Total calcium: 8.9 – 10.1 mg/dl
- Free or ionized calcium: 4.8 – 5.7 mg/dl
- Serum calcium is affected by two main factors – the parathyroid hormone and vitamin D, or, 1, 25 di-hydroxycholecalciferol.
- Hypocalcaemia can occur in hypoparathyroidism or vitamin D deficiency

- Hypercalcemia can occur in hyperparathyroidism, usually associated with malignant tumors of the parathyroid gland.

Magnesium:

- Magnesium is an important intracellular cation that plays an important role in transport, replication, and metabolism.
- Normal range: 0.7 – 1.1 mmol/l
- Abnormal levels of magnesium coexist with other electrolyte imbalances. Patients with renal failure or gastrointestinal disturbances must be monitored for magnesium deficiency.
- Low magnesium levels can cause dangerous arrhythmias, and must be corrected immediately.
- High magnesium levels are not clinically significant, but may be used as a prognostic marker in patients with congestive cardiac failure.

Chloride:

- Chloride is the main anion in the extracellular fluid.
- Like sodium, it also plays an important role in maintaining osmotic balance and acid-base balance, thereby maintaining cellular integrity.
- Normal range: 98 – 106 mmol/l

- Mostly, chloride levels tend to parallel changes in sodium levels in the body, and most conditions that increase or decrease sodium levels will also cause a similar change in chloride levels.

- The exception to this is acid-base disorders where chloride levels change independent of sodium levels. Hypochloremia may be seen in respiratory acidosis, while hyperchloremia may be seen in respiratory alkalosis.

Phosphorous:

- Like calcium, phosphorous also forms an important part of the body's skeleton and plays an important role in bone metabolism.

- Normal range: 2.5 – 4.5 mg/dl

- It is also affected by parathyroid hormone and vitamin D, but the changes are inverse to the changes of serum calcium.

- Hypophosphatemia is seen in vitamin D deficiency and hyperparathyroidism.

- Hyperphosphatemia is seen in hypoparathyroidism.

There are several other electrolytes which are present in small amounts in the body. A summary of other various electrolytes present in the body, their functions and normal levels has been given below:

BOX I: BLOOD VALUES OF ELECTROLYTES

ELECTROLYTE	NORMAL RANGE	SIGNIFICANCE
Ammonia	15 – 50 µmol/l	Breakdown product of most proteins Metabolized by liver into urea Increases in liver disorders
Ceruloplasmin	15 – 60 mg/dl	Copper carrying protein Synthesized by liver Decreased in liver disorders
Copper	70 – 150 µg/dl	Plays a role in iron absorption Aids in RBC formation with iron Incorporated in several metabolic proteins and enzymes
Ferritin	12 – 300 ng/ml (males) 12 – 150 ng/ml	Carrier of iron Marks the total amount of iron in the body

	(females)	
Pyruvate	300 – 900 µg/dl	Product of glucose metabolism Key role in aerobic respiration
Transferrin	65 – 180 µg/dl (males) 30 – 170 µg/dl (females)	Transports iron from duodenum to tissues of the body
Urea	1.2 – 3 mmol/l	Synthesized in liver from ammonia, excretes waste nitrogen from the body through renal system
Uric acid	0.18 – 0.48 mmol/l	Formed by degradation of purines. Normally excreted by kidney; excess accumulation in joints can cause gout.
Zinc	70 – 100 µmol/l	Plays a role in wound healing, cell growth and division.

REFERENCES:

1. George L. Ackerman. Chapter 194. Walker HK, Hall WD, Hurst JW, editors. *Clinical Methods: The History, Physical, and Laboratory Examinations*. 3rd edition. Boston: Butterworths: 1990.

2. Fitzsimons, E. J., & Sendroy, J. (1961). Distribution of electrolytes in human blood. *Journal of Biological Chemistry*, *236*(5), 1595-1601.

3. Laboratory reference range values. Available at http://www.stedmansonline.com/webFiles/Dict-Stedmans28/APP17.pdf.

EXERCISES:

1. The normal range for Potassium for a healthy person is:

        a.   0 – 10

        b.   1.2 - 3.4

        c.   2.7– 4.8

        d.   3.5 – 5.0

2. What is the normal range of chloride?

        a.   15 – 30

        b.   25 – 40

        c.   60 – 85

        d.   95 – 105

3. The normal expected range of sodium seen on lab tests is:

        a.   3.5 – 5

        b.   135 – 145

        c.   120 – 140

        d.   75 – 100

4. What is the normal value of serum calcium?

        a.   9 – 10.5

        b.   98 – 106

        c.   150 – 200

        d.   3.5 – 5

5. Which among the following is a carrier for copper?

    a. Ferritin

    b. Ceruloplasmin

    c. Transferin

    d. Hemoglobin

8. TESTS FOR CARDIAC DISEASE

CARDIAC ENZYMES

The rationale behind the use of cardiac enzymes

- One of the most common medical emergencies that can occur with regard to the cardiac system is a myocardial infarction.

- Myocardial infarction occurs secondary to decreased blood supply to the myocardium of the heart, which causes ischemia.

- This ischemia causes irreversible necrosis of the myocardium, which is referred to as an infarct.

- When the myocardium gets damaged, certain enzymes get released into the blood stream, and are present in increased levels in blood. These are referred to as cardiac enzymes.
- These enzymes are useful clinically as markers to diagnose myocardial infarction, in the presence of suspicious signs of the same.
- There are various such enzymes which are used as cardiac markers, given below:
  - Cardiac troponins
  - Creatine phosphokinase
  - Lactate dehydrogenase
  - Serum glutamic oxaloacetic transaminase
  - Myoglobin
- However, both the European Society of Cardiology and the American College of Cardiology state that the only biomarker that is recommended to be used for the diagnosis of acute MI is cardiac troponin, because it has superior accuracy and sensitivity compared to the others. However, the other markers also have a role in ruling out MI and evaluating additional cardiac muscle injury over time.

Details of the various cardiac enzyme markers are given below:

Cardiac troponins:

- These proteins, found in skeletal and cardiac muscle, have a regulatory function.
- This enzyme has three subunits – troponin –I, troponin – C and troponin – T. Of these, troponin- I and troponin-T are specific to the myocardium.
- Normal value of troponin is< 0.01 ng/ml.
- This enzyme is released in 2 – 4 hours and peaks within 10 – 24 hours of MI. It drops within 1 – 2 weeks.
- Troponins can also be used to calculate the size of the infarct. For this, the values must be measured on the third day.
- However, troponins can also be elevated in pulmonary embolism, myocarditis, and cardiac failure. The laboratory values therefore must be taken in conjunction with clinical signs.

Creatine phosphokinase (CK):

- This enzyme catalyzes the conversion of creatine to creatinine in cells of the heart, skeletal muscle, and brain tissue. Since this is a catabolic process, the levels of this enzyme are also increased in tissue damage.
- Normal value: 25 – 200 U/L

- CK has three isozymes, namely, CK-MM, CK-MB, and CK-BB.

- CK-BB is found in the brain tissue, while CK-MM and CK-MB are found in skeletal and cardiac muscle.

- Of these CK-MB is highly sensitive to myocardial damage.

- It elevates 4 to 6 hours after an acute MI, peaks in 18 to 24 hours, and returns to normal within 3 to 4 days.

- This enzyme has a short duration of increase, and therefore it cannot be used for late diagnosis of acute MI. If the levels rise again, however, it may suggest infarct extension.

- Normal value of CK-MB: 0 – 4 ng/ml

Lactate dehydrogenase (LDH) :

- This enzyme catalyzes the conversion of lactic acid to pyruvic acid, which is an essential step in glucose metabolism.

- Any type of cellular damage tends to increase the levels of this enzyme.

- There are five isozymes of LDH (LDH1, LDH2, LDH3, LDH4 and LDH5). Of these, LDH1 and LDH2 appear in the heart, red blood cells, and kidneys. Therefore, it is these isozymes which are evaluated.

- Normal values: 140 – 280 U/L

- Total LDH level rises 2 – 5 days after an MI. This elevated level lasts for 10 days.

- Total LDH can increase in several conditions. Sometimes, even if the total value is within normal limits, the levels of isozymes may be altered.

- Therefore it is important to check the ratio of the various isozymes.

- Usually LDH-1 forms 17.5% to 28.3% of the total, while LDH-2 forms 30.4% to 36.4% of the total.

- In normal cases, the level of LDH-1 is less than LDH-2 as seen above. However, after an acute MI, the level of LDH-2 does not change but the level of LDH-1 rises. This condition is called a flipped condition.

- This flipped pattern appears 12-24 hours after an MI and remains so for 48 hours.

Serum glutamic oxaloacetic transaminase (Aspartate Transaminase):

- This enzyme, which is present largely in the liver and heart, tends to spike in 8 to 12 hours after an infarction. It reaches a peak in 24 – 48 hours after the infarction.

- It was the first enzyme to be used as a cardiac marker.
- Normal values: 5 – 50 IU/L
- By itself, it is not particularly indicative of MI as serum levels of this enzyme can also increase in other conditions such as liver disease, pancreatitis etc.
- It is, however, used in conjunction with other enzyme results for a more definitive diagnosis of MI.

Myoglobin:

- Myoglobin is a protein which is structurally similar to hemoglobin. It is found in muscle tissue and it is responsible for binding iron and oxygen.
- Although myoglobin is technically not a cardiac enzyme, its levels are used in conjunction with cardiac enzymes to confirm myocardial damage.
- Myoglobin helps to estimate the amount of muscle damage but does not indicate the site of damage, which helps to accurately diagnose an MI.
- Normal values: 30 – 90 ng/ml.
- This protein becomes abnormal within 1 - 2 hours of an MI with a peak in 4 - 8 hours. It drops to normal in 12 - 24 hours.

Pattern of cardiac enzyme levels during myocardial infarction:

- Serum creatine phosphokinase activity goes over the normal range within 6 or 7 hours.

- Reaches a peak within 24 hours, often within 2-10 times the normal range.

- It takes 3 to 4 days to subside to normal levels.

- The serum LDH activity exceeds normal activity within 24 to 48 hours.

- Peaks within 3 to 6 days.

- The serum SGOT (serum glutamic oxaloacetic transaminase), which is released into the blood stream when the liver or the heart is damaged, and serum glutamic pyruvic transaminase (SGPT) also help in determining abnormal cardiac states.

- Troponin I and Troponin T spike over the first day and remain elevated for 6 or 7 days.

  This has been summarized in the table below.

BOX 1. CARDIAC ENZYME PATTERNS IN MYOCARDIAL INFARCTION			
MI Serum Markers	Detected (Hours)	Peak (Hours)	Fall (Hours)
Myoglobin	1 – 3	1 – 8	12 – 18
CK/CK-MB	3 – 8	12 – 16	24 – 48
MB Isoforms	1 – 6	4 – 8	12 – 48
Troponin Complex	3 – 6	10 – 24	cTn I: 5 – 9 days cTn T: 7 – 14 days

LIPID PROFILE AND LABORATORY VALUES

This Panel evaluates the levels of different lipids that are present in our body. Lipids or fats have several important functions in the body. They play a role in producing hormones, absorption of nutrients from the digestive tract, and serve as a source of energy. Although this test is referred to as 'lipid' profile, this test detects the levels of two actual lipids (cholesterol and triglyceride) and three lipoproteins. The different components evaluated in the panel are as follows:

Low density lipoprotein:

- LDL, also referred to as the 'bad fat', transports cholesterol from the liver, where it is formed, to the various cells of the body.

- There is a direct positive correlation between high LDL levels and the incidence of arterial atherosclerosis.

High density lipoprotein:

- HDL is also referred to as the 'good fat', because it transports cholesterol from the cells and tissues back to the liver, thereby preventing excess blood levels of these components.

- HDL clears cholesterol from the blood vessel wall, thereby preventing atherosclerotic narrowing of blood vessels.

- High HDL levels are generally indicative of a healthy lifestyle, except in the case of liver disease.

Triglycerides:

- The body stores fat in the form of triglycerides.
- Whenever lipids are needed for energy, they are broken down from triglycerides.
- High levels show the presence of one of the following diseases:
    o Hypothyroidism
    o Myocardial infarction
    o Nephrotic syndrome
    o Liver disease
    o Metabolic disorders
    o Atherosclerosis
    o Pancreatitis
    o Toxemia.

Total cholesterol:

- Cholesterol, although implicated in cardiovascular disorders, has several essential functions:
    o They form an integral part of the cell wall
    o Play an important role in the production of steroid hormones in the body

- o Help in the activation of vitamin D when exposed to sunlight
- o Are involved in the production of bile, which is essential to the digestion process.
- Elevated cholesterol occurs during hypothyroidism, atherosclerosis, pregnancy, and diabetes.
- Low levels are seen during anemia, malignancies, liver insufficiency, malnutrition, and depression

Very low density lipoprotein (VLDL):

- VLDL serves as the body's internal transport system for lipids.
- It transports cholesterol and triglycerides within the body.

Cholesterol: HDL ratio:

- Total cholesterol includes the fat contained in LDL, HDL, as well as triglycerides.
- The cholesterol: HDL ratio tells us the amount of HDL that is part of the total cholesterol.
- It is calculated by dividing the total cholesterol level by the HDL level of a patient.
- If this ratio is high, it indicates increase risk of developing atherosclerotic diseases.

A summary of the normal values and optimum value of the various components of the lipid profile is detailed below:

BOX 2. LABORATORY VALUES FOR LIPID PROFILE		
	NORMAL RANGE	**OPTIMAL READING**
CHOLESTEROL	120 – 240 mg/dl	180
LOW DENSITY LIPOPROTEIN (LDL)	62 – 130 mg/dl	81
HIGH DENSITY LIPOPROTEIN (HDL)	35 – 135 mg/dl	+85 mg/dl
TRIGLYCERIDES	0 – 200 mg/dl	100
CHOLESTEROL/LDL RATIO	1 – 6	3.5

REFERENCES:

1. Guideline. Amsterdam EA, Wenger NK, Brindis RG, et al, for the ACC/AHA Task Force Members. 2014 AHA/ACC guideline for the management of patients with non-ST-elevation acute coronary syndromes: a report of the American College of Cardiology/American Heart Association Task Force on Practice Guidelines. *Circulation.* 2014 Dec 23. 130 (25):e344-426.

2. Christenson RH; Ohman EM; Topol EJ; et al. (September 1997). "Assessment of coronary reperfusion after thrombolysis with a model combining myoglobin, creatine kinase-MB, and clinical variables. TAMI-7 Study Group. Thrombolysis and Angioplasty in Myocardial Infarction-7". *Circulation.* 96 (6): 1776–82. doi:10.1161/01.cir.96.6.1776. PMID 9323061.

3. Reichlin, T., Hochholzer, W., Bassetti, S., Steuer, S., Stelzig, C., Hartwiger, S., ... & Noveanu, M. (2009). Early diagnosis of myocardial infarction with sensitive cardiac troponin assays. *New England Journal of Medicine, 361*(9), 858-867.

4. Miller M, Stone NJ, Ballantyne C, et al. Triglycerides and cardiovascular disease: a scientific statement from the American Heart Association. *Circulation.* 2011 May 24. 123(20):2292-333.

5. Ayaz K., M., & Ahsan, M. (2016). Evaluation and Interpretation of Lipid Profile Based on the National Cholesterol Education Programme Adult Treatment Panel III Guidelines. *Indian Journal Of Medical & Health Sciences*, *3*(2), 123-129. http://dx.doi.org/10.21088/ijmhs.2347.9981.3216.9

EXERCISES:

1. Which of the following cardiac markers is the most sensitive to diagnose a myocardial infarction?
    a. Creatine Phosphokinase
    b. Cardiac troponins
    c. Lactate dehydrogenase
    d. Aspartate aminotransferase

2. Which of the following enzymes is not a cardiac marker for myocardial infarction?
    a. Myoglobin
    b. Creatinine Phosphokinase
    c. Troponin
    d. Acid phosphatase

3. What is the normal level of Creatinine phosphokinase in a healthy adult?
    a. 25 – 200 U/l
    b. 15 – 100 U/l
    c. 35 – 300 U/l
    d. 45 – 150 U/l

4. Which of the following values indicates that the patient is at risk of atherosclerotic disease?
    a. Triglycerides : 150 mg/dl

b. HDL: 120 mg/dl

c. LDL: 180 mg/dl

d. Cholesterol: 150 mg/dl

5. Which of the following lipids is considered healthy when the value increases?

    a. Very Low Density Lipoprotein

    b. Low Density Lipoprotein

    c. High Density Lipoprotein

    d. Total Cholesterol

9. SPECIFIC TESTS FOR INFECTION-SEROLOGICAL TESTS

When an infection invades the body, antibodies are produced as a defense mechanism against the micro-organisms. Serological tests are used to assess the values of these antibodies that are present in the blood. Serological tests can be used for a wide variety of diseases.

The interpretation of serological test results is fairly simple for a nurse. If the test indicates that no antibodies are present, there is no infection. If there are antibodies present, it could indicate a current infection, past infection, or sometimes, presence of an autoimmune disease. The results must always be correlated with clinical findings.

While discussing all the serological tests is beyond the scope of this book, the most important ones required for nurses are outlined in this chapter.

Tests for HIV:

- The human immunodeficiency virus causes a disease called AIDS (Acquired immune deficiency syndrome).

- Antibodies to HIV will develop in 90-95% individuals within three months of exposure, and will develop in 99% individuals within six months of exposure.

- There are two serological tests for HIV. The ELISA test is generally used for screening purposes while the Western blot test is a confirmatory test.

- A reference value of less than 1.0 is considered negative.

- Any patient who tests positive for HIV will need more laboratory testing, due to the extremely debilitating nature of the disease.

- The following tests need to be performed in these patients: CD4 count:

- The HIV virus tends to destroy the CD4 T-cells, so it is important to periodically review the count of these cells.

- The normal range of CD4 cells in a healthy body: 500 cells per cubic mm of blood.

- A count lower than $200/mm^3$ is diagnosed as AIDS.

- CD4 percentage, which determines the ratio of these cells to total white blood cells, gives a more accurate picture.

Viral load test

- Measures the number of virus particles per milliliter of blood.
- A viral load below 50 is said to be undetectable.
- Once a patient starts anti-retroviral therapy, this value is used to monitor the patient's response to treatment.

Tests for Hepatitis B:

- There are several serological markers for hepatitis B infection. These include HBsAg, anti-HBs, HBeAg, anti-HBe, and anti-HBc.
- HBsAg is the main serological marker for hepatitis B infection. It appears in the serum 1 to 10 weeks after exposure, and persists for more than six months.
- Anti-Hbs is detected in patients who have undergone immunization.

Test for typhoid: Widal test

- This test tests two different types of antibodies – H-agglutinin and O-agglutinin
- H-agglutinin tests past infection while O-agglutinin tests active infection.
- A titer of more than 1:160 is considered to be positive.

Other tests:

- Bacterial infections such as:
    - Brucellosis
    - Syphilis
- Viruses such as :
    - Measles
    - Rubella
    - Cytomegalovirus and herpes virus
- Fungal infections such as aspergillosis
- Parasite infections such as amoebiasis

BACTEREMIA AND SEPTIC SHOCK WORKUP:

In the antibiotic era, most infections are not life threatening. However, in rare cases, micro-organisms can enter the bloodstream and can threaten host defenses

The following tests are done when bacteremia or septic shock is suspected:

- Complete blood count: including hemoglobin, white blood cell count, and differential count. WBC of more than 15 per histopathological field is indicative of bacteremia.
- Platelet count, along with PT and APTT is very important to monitor disseminated intravascular coagulation.

- Serum electrolytes to assess for dehydration and acidosis.

- Glucose to monitor for hyperglycemia.

- Renal functions and liver function tests.

REFERENCES:

1. Song JE, Kim DY. Diagnosis of hepatitis B. *Annals of Translational Medicine.* 2016;4(18):338. doi:10.21037/atm.2016.09.11

2. Kao, J. (2008). Diagnosis of hepatitis B virus infection through serological and virological markers. *Expert Review of Gastroenterology & Hepatology*, 2(4), pp.553-562.

3. Specimens for Serological Tests. (1950). *BMJ*, 1(4648), pp.301-302..

4. Pang T, Puthucheary SD. Significance and value of the Widal test in the diagnosis of typhoid fever in an endemic area. *Journal of Clinical Pathology.* 1983;36(4):471-475.

5. Mole, R. (1948). The diagnostic value of the widal test in the inoculated. *Journal of Hygiene*, 46(01), pp.98-100.

EXERCISES:

1. Which of the following sexually transmitted diseases are not curable?

    a. Gonorrhea

    b. Syphilis

    c. Hepatitis B

    d. Chlamydia

2. In a patient who is 7 years old, which of the following cell counts of CD4 indicates that he or she has HIV infection?

    a. 650 cells per micro liter of blood

    b. 180 cells per micro liter of blood

    c. 400 cells per micro liter of blood

    d. 500 cells per micro liter of blood

3. If the anti retroviral therapy is effective, what would be the expected viral load?

    a. 50 particles per ml

    b. 100 particles per ml

    c. 150 particles per ml

    d. 200 particles per ml

4. What lower limit of white blood cells per histopathological field is indicative of bacteremia?

    a. 10

      b. 15

      c. 20

      d. 25

5. Which panel of tests helps to monitor for Disseminated Intravascular Coagulation in septic shock?

      a. Liver function panel

      b. Renal function panel

      c. Coagulation panel

      d. Glucose panel

10. TESTS FOR MALIGNANT CONDITIONS– TUMOR MARKERS

Tumor markers are usually soluble glycoproteins that are usually produced by tumor cells. Therefore, they increase in concentration in the bloodstream when various types of cancers are present. This is used clinically to diagnose and evaluate cancers. The role of tumor markers in cancer diagnosis are as follows:

- To screen patients for presence or absence of malignancy.
- To diagnose specific tumor types, in case biopsy is not feasible.
- For staging the tumor and evaluating prognosis.

- To monitor patients who have undergone treatment for cancer, both to monitor the effectiveness of treatment, and to detect recurrences.

Tumor markers can also increase in concentration under certain benign conditions, which limits their usefulness. Various tumor markers differ in their usefulness for the above purposes. The important types of tumor markers that are currently in use are described below:

Alpha fetoprotein:

- This is a protein that is synthesized by the liver in early fetal life, and is therefore normally present in the blood during pregnancy. However, it reduces soon after birth.
- Normal value: 0 – 44 ng/ml
- Elevated levels of alpha fetoprotein are associated with:
  - Liver tumors – hepatocellular carcinoma and hepatoblastoma
  - Tumors of the ovary and testes.

Beta human chorionic gonadotropin:

- This protein is normally produced by the placenta.
- Beta-hcg is most commonly increased in pregnancy.
- However, it is also increased in the presence of gynecological tumors such as :
  - Choriocarcinoma of the uterus

- o Embryonal carcinomas
- o Dysgerminomas
- o Mixed cell tumors
- Normal value: < 5 IU/l

Cancer Antigen 19 - 9:

- This is a glycoprotein antigen that is present in the epithelial cells of the pancreas, cells of the biliary duct, salivary glands, endometrium, stomach, gall bladder, and colon.
- Normal value: < 40 U/ml
- It can be increased in benign conditions affecting the above cells such as inflammatory bowel disease, pancreatitis, cholangitis, biliary tract obstruction etc.
- It tends to be increased in the following malignancies: pancreatic cancers, hepatocellular cancers, bile duct cancers, esophageal and gastric cancers, and ovarian cancers.
- This antigen alone, however, is not sensitive enough for screening for these cancers.
- It may be used to determine the extent and prognosis, in conjunction with other methods.
- It is, however, useful as a marker to detect recurrences.

Carcinoembryonic antigen (CEA)

- This glycoprotein is produced by cells of the gastrointestinal tract during embryonic development, and very minimal amounts are found in the human body after birth.
- Normal value: $< 4\mu g/l$
- Malignancies which cause increased CEA are cancers of the colon and rectum, and less commonly, cancers of the pancreas, stomach, lung, breast, thyroid gland, and ovaries.
- Elevation of this marker is also found in certain benign conditions such as smoking, inflammatory bowel disease, pancreatitis, cirrhosis, and benign tumors.
- Because of its low sensitivity and specificity, it is used for monitoring rather than for screening and diagnosis.

Prostatic acid phosphatase:

- Acid phosphatase is a liver enzyme that is present in low concentrations in serum.
- Normal value is 2 ng/ml or less, or $0 - 3$ U/dl
- Acid phosphatase is largely used as a marker for detecting and assessing the prognosis of prostate cancers.
- Its levels are highly increased in prostate cancer, benign prostate hypertrophy, or prostate infarction

- This enzyme will show moderate increase in Paget's disease, hyperparathyroidism, sickle cell disease, multiple myeloma, and lysosomal diseases.

Prostate specific antigen (PSA):

- This is a proteolytic enzyme released by epithelial cells of the prostate gland. Its function is to break down high molecular weight proteins in order to liquefy semen.
- Normal value: $< 4\mu g/l$
- It may be used with other tests to screen patients for prostate cancer, and to confirm if prostate cancer is present.
- It may also be slightly increased in prostatitis or benign prostate hypertrophy.

There are several other proteins that are used as tumor markers. Although the list is exhaustive, a few distinct markers have been summarized in the box below:

BOX 1. SUMMARY OF VARIOUS TUMOR MARKERS	
TUMOR MARKER	MALIGNANCY IN WHICH IT IS RAISED
CA 15 3	Breast cancer
CA 27 29	Breast cancer

CA 125	Ovarian cancer
Calcitonin	Medullary thyroid carcinoma
Calretinin	Mesothelioma
Chromosomes 3, 7, 17, and 9p21	Bladder cancer
Desmin	Smooth and skeletal muscle sarcomas
Epithelium membrane antigen	Carcinomas and sarcomas
Factor VIII, CD 31	Vascular sarcoma
Glial fibrillary acidic protein	Glioma
Immunoglobulins	Lymphoma, leukemia
Keratins	Carcinomas, sarcomas
MART 1	Melanomas, steroid producing tumors
MSA (Muscle specific actin)	Myosarcomas
Neurofilaments, neuronspecific enolase	Neuroendocrine tumors
Placental alkaline phosphatase	Seminoma, dysgerminoma
S-100 protein	Melanomas, sarcomas

Synaptophysin	Neuroendocrine tumors
Vimentin	Sarcoma, renal and lung carcinomas

REFERENCES:

1. Sturgeon CM, Duffy MJ, Stenman UH, et al: National Academy of Clinical Biochemistry laboratory medicine practice guidelines for use of tumor markers in testicular, prostate, colorectal, breast, and ovarian cancers. Clin Chem 2008 Dec; 54(12):e11-79

2. Cidón, E. and Bustamante, R. (2010). Gastric Cancer: Tumor Markers as Predictive Factors for Preoperative Staging. *Journal of Gastrointestinal Cancer*, 42(3), pp.127-130.

3. The value of tumor markers in the diagnosis, staging and prognosis of lung cancer. (1996). *Lung Cancer*, 14(2-3), p.395.

4. Hansen, H. J., Snyder, J. J., Miller, E., Vandevoorde, J. P., Miller, O. N., Hines, L. R., & Burns, J. J. (1974). Carcinoembryonic antigen (CEA) assay: A laboratory adjunct in the diagnosis and management of cancer. *Human Pathology*, 5(2), 139-147.

5. Bull H, Murray PG, Thomas D, Fraser AM, Nelson PN. Acid phosphatases. *Molecular Pathology*. 2002;55(2):65-72.

EXERCISES:

1. Which of the following tumors is not associated with beta human chorionic gonadotropin?

    a. Choriocarcinomas

    b. Prostatic carcinomas

    c. Dysgeminomas

    d. Mixed cell tumors

2. What is the normal reference range for alpha fetoprotein?

    a. 5 – 15 ng/ml

    b. 0 – 44 ng/ml

    c. 6 – 30 ng/ml

    d. 15 – 25 ng/ml

3. Which of the following tumor markers are associated with pancreatic cancer?

    a. Cancer Antigen 19 9

    b. Cancer Antigen 15 3

    c. Cancer Antigen 27 29

    d. Cancer Antigen 125

4. Which of the following is not used as a tumor marker?

    a. Cytokeratin

    b. Desmin

    c. Vimentin

    d. Collagen

5. S-100 protein increase is associated with which of the following conditions?

    a. Sarcomas

    b. Melanomas

    c. Carcinomas

    d. Both a and b

11. TESTS FOR MISCELLANEOUS CONDITIONS

Alpha – 1 antitrypsin:

- This enzyme inhibits tissue damage that is caused by trypsin, elastin, and other proteases.
- Normal values: 20 – 50 μmol/l
- Alpha-1 antitrypsin deficiency may be congenital. It is associated with the development of early-onset emphysema, and neonatal hepatitis, which may progress to cirrhosis.
- Any inflammatory process in the body can cause increased levels of this enzyme.

Angiotensin converting enzyme:

- This enzyme plays a role in vasoconstriction, by helping rennin from the kidneys convert into angiotensin. It therefore results in vasoconstriction and increased blood pressure.
- Normal value: 23 – 57 U/l
- The levels of this enzyme may be increased in sarcoidosis, Gaucher's disease, hyperthyroidism, psoriasis, amyloidosis, and histoplasmosis.
- Increased levels of this enzyme is used for diagnosing sarcoidosis, in combination with other modalities like radiology and histopathology

C- reactive protein:

- This is an acute phase serum protein that plays an important role in infection and inflammation.
- Normal value: < 5mg/ml, but it increases 100-1000 fold during inflammation or trauma.
- This test is done whenever inflammatory process is suspected in the body e.g., autoimmune diseases, systemic lupus erythematosus.
- This test can be combined with ESR, to rule out inflammatory causes for ESR increase.
- Serial tests of this protein are also done in order to monitor ongoing inflammatory process.

Erythrocyte sedimentation rate (ESR):

- Erythrocyte sedimentation rate shows how much inflammation is present in the body. This test measures the speed at which RBC fall to the bottom of a test tube.
- This test is indicated in:
  - o Muscle contractions
  - o Unexplained fevers
  - o Unexplained vague symptoms
  - o Certain types of arthritis

- Normal range varies depending on the method, age, and sex. According to the *Westergren method:*
  - o <u>Adults:</u>
    - Men aged less than 50 years: lower than 15 mm/hr.
    - Men older than 50 years of age: lower than 20 mm/hr.
    - Women aged less than 50 years: lower than 20 mm/hr.
    - Women older than 50 years: lower than 30 mm/hr.
  - o <u>Children</u>
    - Newborn: $0 - 2$ mm/hr.
    - Newborn to puberty: $3 - 13$ mm/hr.

- This test can use be used to track bone infections, inflammatory diseases, autoimmune disorders, some types of arthritis and tissue death

- Though the result is indicative, it is not conclusive regarding diagnosis. One has to confirm the diagnosis through other tests. Medical conditions linked to abnormal results include kidney disease, anemia, pregnancy, cancers, thyroid disease etc.

- People with autoimmune disorders have a higher incidence of increased ESR. Common examples include lupus and rheumatoid arthritis. Other examples are primary macroglobulinemia, allergic vasculitis, hyperfibrinogenemia, polymyalgia rheumatica, giant cell arteritis, and necrotizing vasculitis.

- Abnormalities in the ESR rates could arise from other conditions. Increased rates may occur due to bone infections, rheumatic fever, tuberculosis, systemic infection, heart or heart valve infections, and severe skin infections. Lower rates can occur in the presence of hyperviscosity, congestive heart failure, sickle cell anemia, or leukemia.

Rheumatoid factor:

- This is an autoantibody produced in rheumatoid arthritis.
- Normal value: < 25 IU/l
- The blood level of this is increased in rheumatoid arthritis, and therefore this test is used for the diagnosis of this autoimmune disease.
- Very high levels of this factor indicate a more aggressive disease.
- The blood levels can be monitored in patients with known rheumatoid arthritis in order to guide treatment protocols.

Markers for muscular dystrophy:

Patients with muscular dystrophy often show abnormal elevations in the following markers:

a) Lactic dehydrogenase
b) Aldolase
c) Phosphohexose isomerase
d) Glutamic-oxalacetic transaminase

This kind of elevation of the enzyme activity is common in those with acute cerebral vascular accidents, but not found in other neurological disorders.

REFERENCES:

1. Greene DN, Elliott-Jelf MC, Straseski JA, Grenache DG. Facilitating the laboratory diagnosis of a1-antitrypsin deficiency. *Am J Clin Pathol*. 2013 Feb. 139(2):184-91

2. Pepys MB, Hirschfield GM. C-reactive protein: a critical update. *J Clin Invest*. 2003 Jun. 111(12):1805-12

3. Firestein, Gary S., et al. *Kelley's Textbook of Rheumatology, Ninth Edition*. China: Elsevier Health, 2012.

4. Pribush, A., Hatskelzon, L. And Meyerstein, N. (2010). A novel approach for assessments of erythrocyte sedimentation rate. *International Journal of Laboratory Hematology*, 33(3), pp.251-257.

5. Walton, J. (2008). Current Research in Muscular Dystrophy A Muscular Dystrophy Group Symposium. *Developmental Medicine & Child Neurology*, 7(2), pp.205-208.

EXERCISES:

1. Alpha – 1 antitrypsin deficiency can result in all the following conditions except:
   a. Emphysema
   b. Hepatitis
   c. Cirrhosis
   d. Inflammation

2. Which of the following ranges approximately indicates the normal range of Angiotensin Converting Enzyme?
   a. 3 – 23 U/l
   b. 23 – 53 U/l
   c. 53 – 73 U/l
   d. 73 – 93 U/l

3. Which of the following conditions is not associated with an increase in Erythrocyte sedimentation rate?
   a. Systemic Lupus Erythematosus
   b. Anemia
   c. Congestive cardiac failure
   d. Pregnancy

4. Which of the following represents a normal Erythrocyte Sedimentation Rate in a young, healthy adult male?
   a. <15 mm/hr

b. <20 mm/hr

c. <25 mm/hr

d. <30 mm/hr

5. One of the following is not a marker for muscular dystrophy:

   a. Serum glutamic oxaloacetic aminotransferase

   b. Lactate dehydrogenase

   c. Acid phosphatase

   d. Aldolase

12. ARTERIAL BLOOD GAS ANALYSIS

Arterial blood gas studies basically evaluate the amount of gases – oxygen and carbon dioxide, in the patient's blood. Assessing this helps to determine the efficacy of respiratory, metabolic, and renal functions of the body. There are five components of arterial blood gases, which are as follows:

Partial pressure of oxygen (PaO2):

- This value indicates the pressure, or amount of oxygen dissolved in the arterial blood.
- This reflects how well the oxygen is able to move from the alveoli of the lungs into the blood stream in order to reach the tissues.

Partial pressure of carbon dioxide (PaCO2):

- This value indicates the amount of carbon dioxide dissolved in the blood.

- This is a reflection of how well carbon dioxide exits the blood and moves out of the body through the lung alveoli.

pH:

- This value measures the acid-base balance of the blood.

- Blood is always slightly basic and has a pH of 7.35 to 7.45.

- If this value decreases, the patient may have acidosis, while, if it increases, the patient may have alkalosis.

Bicarbonate (HCO3):

- Bicarbonate is a compound that is naturally present in the blood.

- It acts as a buffer and maintains the blood at homeostatic pH.

Oxygen saturation (SaO2):

- This value evaluates the proportion of hemoglobin in the blood that is currently carrying oxygen.

- Although this also evaluates the amount of oxygen in the blood, while PaO2 measures the concentration of oxygen in plasma. This value basically measures the concentration of oxygen in hemoglobin.

A summary of the normal ranges of arterial blood gas components is listed below.

BOX 1. NORMAL VALUES OF ARTERIAL BLOOD GAS COMPONENTS	
COMPONENT MEASURED IN ARTERIAL BLOOD	NORMAL RANGE
Partial pressure of oxygen (PaO2)	80 – 100 mmHg
Partial pressure of carbon dioxide (PaCO2)	35 – 45 mmHg
Arterial blood Ph	7.35 – 7.45
Oxygen saturation (SaO2)	95 – 100%
Bicarbonate (HCO3)	22 – 26 mEq/l

In order to correctly diagnose diseases, serial ABGs may usually be taken. It is important to remember that, in a normal ABG:

- pH and PaCO2 move in opposite directions
- HCO3 and PaCO2 move in the same direction.

Using arterial blood gases to evaluate acid-base disorders:

- ABG is primarily used to evaluate acid-base disorders. Acid-base disorders may be metabolic, respiratory, or mixed disorders. Abnormal values on an ABG would indicate one of these disorders. The following points must be kept in mind while trying to interpret acid-base disorders:

- A low pH indicates acidosis while a high pH indicates alkalosis.

- Change in PaCO2 levels is indicative of a respiratory problem while change in HCO3 is indicative of a metabolic problem.

- The acronym ROME (Respiratory Opposite, Metabolic Equal) is worth remembering here.

- If the pH and pCO2 move in opposite directions(one value increases from normal while the other decreases, or vice-versa), then the primary problem is respiratory.

- If both pH and HCO3 move in the same direction, (both values are higher, and both are lower than normal), then the primary problem is metabolic.

- In uncompensated disorders, the HCO3 remains normal for respiratory disorders while PaCO2 remains normal for metabolic disorders.

- However, usually the body tries to compensate for the abnormal blood pH by attempting to correct it.

- o In respiratory disorders, compensation is done by the kidneys, which tend to retain more bicarbonate in acidosis (increasing blood HCO3), and excrete more bicarbonate in alkalosis (decreased blood HCO3).
- o In metabolic disorders, the compensation is done by the lungs, which tries to excrete carbon dioxide in acidosis (low PaCO2), and tries to retain it in alkalosis (high PaCO2).

- Anion Gap: Anion Gap is the difference between the primary measured cations (Na+, K+) and anions (Cl⁻, HCO3⁻) that are present in the blood.
  - o $AG = (Na^+ + K^+) - (Cl^- - HCO3^-)$
  - o Normal AG is 3 – 11 mEq/l
  - o A high anion gap, especially over 20 mEq/l, may be indicative of metabolic acidosis.

The values of various components of ABG in acid-base disorders are given below:

BOX 2. ABG VALUES IN ACID-BASE DISORDERS			
	PaCO2	pH	HCO3
Metabolic acidosis	Normal 35 – 45 mmHg	< 7.35	< 22 mmol/l
Metabolic alkalosis	Normal 35 – 45 mmHg	> 7.45	> 26 mmol/l
Respiratory acidosis	> 45mmHg	< 7.35	Normal 22 – 26 mEq/l
Respiratory alkalosis	< 35 mmHg	> 7.45	Normal 22 – 26 mEq/l
Compensated metabolic acidosis	< 35 mmHg	< 7.35	< 22 mmol/l
Compensated metabolic alkalosis	> 45 mmHg	>7.45	> 26 mmol/l

Compensated respiratory acidosis	> 45mmHg	< 7.35	> 26 mmol/l
Compensated respiratory alkalosis	< 35 mmHg	>7.45	< 22 mmol/l

REFERENCES:

1. Sood P, Paul G, Puri S. Interpretation of arterial blood gas. *Indian Journal of Critical Care Medicine: Peer-reviewed, Official Publication of Indian Society of Critical Care Medicine.* 2010;14(2):57-64. doi:10.4103/0972-5229.68215.

2. Woodrow, P. (2004). Arterial blood gas analysis. *Nursing standard, 18*(21), 45-52.

3. Rubio, M. (1987). Arterial Blood Gas Analysis. *Annals Of Internal Medicine, 106*(3), 474. http://dx.doi.org/10.7326/0003-4819-106-3-474_2

4. Stein, P. D., Goldhaber, S. Z., Henry, J. W., & Miller, A. C. (1996). Arterial blood gas analysis in the assessment of suspected acute pulmonary embolism. *Chest, 109*(1), 78-81.

EXERCISES:

1. The normal value of pH of the blood is
    a. 7.53
    b. 7.64
    c. 7.35
    d. 7.28

2. Which   of these is the respiratory parameter of the arterial blood gas?
    a. PaO2
    b. PaCO2
    c. HCO3
    d. SaO2

3. Interpret the underlying acid – base disorder for the following blood gas parameters: pH - 7.33; PaCO2 – 40; HCO3 – 21
    a. Uncompensated respiratory acidosis
    b. Partially compensated respiratory acidosis
    c. Uncompensated metabolic acidosis
    d. Partially compensated metabolic acidosis

4. If the respiratory rate increases after a long standing metabolic acidosis, this is an example of:
    a. Mixed acidosis

b. Primary respiratory disorder

c. Compensation

d. Anion gap

5. Interpret the underlying acid – base disorder from the following blood gas parameters: pH - 7.62; PaCO2 – 30; HCO3 – 20

    a. Uncompensated respiratory alkalosis

    b. Partially compensated respiratory alkalosis

    c. Uncompensated metabolic alkalosis

    d. Partially compensated metabolic alkalosis

13. BODY FLUID AND STOOL ANALYSIS

URINE ANALYSIS

Routine urine analysis is always done as a part of regular medical examination or prior to surgery. Urine analysis is useful as a screening tool for both renal and systemic pathologies. The method of obtaining a proper urine specimen has been described in Chapter 1.

The following tests are done as a part of routine urine analysis

GROSS VISUAL EXAMINATION:

Color and appearance:

- Normal color of urine is yellow, owing to the presence of a pigment called urochrome. This can vary from pale, straw-colored, to a dark or deep amber color, depending on the concentration.

- Urine color can change due to certain foods, drugs, or medical conditions. These have been outlined in Box 1.

BOX 1. CAUSES OF CHANGE IN URINE COLOR			
COLOR OF URINE	MEDICAL CONDITIONS	DRUGS	FOODS
Red	Hemoglobinurea Porphyrias Nephrolithiasis Urinary tract infections	Chlorpromazine Thioridazine	Beets Blackberries
Orange	--	Rifampicicn Phenzopyridine	Carrots Vitamin C rich foods
Blue	Tryptophan malabsorption	Methylene blue Indomethacin Amitriptyline	--

Purple	Bactiurea – in patients with indwelling catheters	--	--
Green	Urinary tract infection	Vitamin B Propofol	Asparagus
Brown	Hepatobiliary disease Gilbert syndrome Tyrosinemia	Metronidazole Levodopa Nitrofurantoin Chloroquine	Fava beans
Black	Alkaptonuria Malignant melanoma	--	--
White	Chyluria Pyuria Phosphate crystals	Propofol	--

- Appearance: The clarity of urine is described as being clear, mildly cloudy, cloudy, or turbid.
- The turbidity increases with increase in urine substances such as cellular debris, crystals, casts, proteins, or bacteria.

Odor/Smell:

- Normal urine has a "nutty" smell.
- A fruity smell is indicative of presence of ketone bodies, which may be seen in uncontrolled diabetes, starvation, or dehydration.
- Fetid odor may be indicative of infection, particularly with E.coli.
- Maple syrup urine disease has sweet smelling urine.
- Phenylketonuria is characterized by a mousy or musty odor.

pH (potential hydrogen):

- Normal urine has a pH of 4.5 – 8.0.
- Acidic urine is seen if patients have uric acid or cystine calculi. It may also be seen in aspirin overdose, uncontrolled diabetes, starvation or dehydration.
- Alkaline urine is seen in patients with renal calculi made of calcium phosphate or magnesium-ammonium phosphate. High levels of pH can also occur if the person has a urinary

tract infection, asthma, a kidney disease or has had severe vomiting.

Specific gravity:

- Specific gravity measures urine concentration and it is therefore a reflection of the kidney's ability to concentrate urine. It may also reflect the patient's hydration status, but this is not always accurate.
- Normal urine has a specific gravity of 1.005 – 1.025.
- High levels occur due to decreased fluid intake or loss of fluid due to vomiting or sweat. It can also occur in nephritic syndrome, glomerulonephritis, liver or heart failure.
- Low levels can indicate too much fluid intake. It can also occur in acute tubular necrosis, pyelonephritis, and diabetes insipidus.

Glucose:

- Ideally, there should be no glucose or trace amounts (1 – 15 mg/dl) present in urine.
- If the blood glucose exceeds 180 mg/dl, the proximal tubules of the kidney cannot reabsorb such large amounts of glucose, and therefore excrete it into the urine.
- This is usually seen in diabetes mellitus, but can also occur in other conditions of impaired tolerance, such as pregnancy.

Ketones:

- The three ketones are acetone, acetoacetic acid, and beta-hydroxy butyric acid. These are produced in the body only when there is fat metabolism, and then they get excreted in urine.

- Under normal conditions, there should be no ketones present in urine.

- Ketones are produced and excreted in starvation or diet-related disorders. Ketones are also found in patients with uncontrolled diabetes.

Protein:

- The amount of protein in urine must be less than 150 mg/dl.
- The presence of protein can indicate diabetes, high blood pressure, leukemia, poison, heart failure, or an infection.
- There are two methods of testing for protein in the urine – the dipstick method and sulfosalicylic acid method
- The dipstick method tests only albumins. It is highly specific, but not sensitive, especially to proteins of a smaller size, e.g. microalbumins. The results of a dipstick may be quantified as:
  - Trace proteinuria: 10 – 30 mg/dl
  - 1+ : 30 mg/dl
  - 2+ : 100 mg/dl

- o 3+ : 300 mg/dl
- o 4+ : 1000mg/dl or more
- Sulfosalicylic acid test (SSA) tests all types of proteins, including globulins, and Bence-Jones protein. The results are quantified as:
  - o 0 : no turbidity, 0 mg/dl
  - o Traces : slight turbidity, 20 mg/dl
  - o 1+ : print visible through specimen, 50 mg/dl
  - o 2+ : print invisible, 200 mg/dl
  - o 3+ : flocculation, 500 mg/dl
  - o 4+ : dense precipitate, 1000 mg/dl or more.
- Patients with proteinuria must be evaluated further to identify the cause.

Nitrites:

- If certain bacteria are present in the urine, they will convert urinary nitrates into nitrites. This is a sensitive test for detecting urinary tract infections.
- Normal urine should test negative for nitrites.
- Not all bacteria can convert nitrates into nitrites (e.g. Staphylococcus, Streptococcus), and therefore a negative result does not rule out the possibility of UTI.

Bilirubin:

- Normal urine should test negative for bilirubin.
- Conjugated or water soluble bilirubin might be excreted in liver diseases such as hepatitis, or in obstructive hepatobiliary conditions.

Urobilirubin:

- Bilirubin is generally converted by bacteria in the intestine to urobilinogen, which is then excreted as urobilirubin.
- The amount of urobilirubin present in normal urine is 0.5 to 1 mg/dl.
- This may be increased in liver diseases or in excessive hemolysis.
- It may be decreased in obstructive biliary disease and cholestasis.

Leukocyte esterase:

- This is an enzyme that is released when white blood cells undergo lysis. Normally, very few WBCs are present in the urine.
- Therefore, normal urine should test negative for leukocyte esterase.
- A positive test is referred to as pyuria which is usually seen in urinary tract infections. This is useful to diagnose UTIs

that are caused by mico-organisms that are difficult to grow in standard urine culture, e.g. Chlamydia, Mycobacteria.

Human chorionic gonadotropin (hCG)

- This is a hormone that is normally produced by the placenta during pregnancy, and is therefore tested only in women.
- If the patient is a man, a note must be made on the chart by using the term NA or "Not Applicable".
- This hormone can be detected in the urine approximately ten days after pregnancy.

MICROSCOPIC ANALYSIS:

The urine sediment is examined for red blood cells, white blood cells, cast, bacteria or yeast cells, squamous cells, and crystals.

Leukocytes (White blood cells):

- There should be less than 2 to 5 WBCs per hpf.
- Abnormal presence shows past or present infection, or contamination of the specimen.
- Urinary eosnophils may indicate acute interstitial nephritis.
- Urinary lymphocytes may indicate tubulointerstitial renal diseases.

Red Blood Cells:

- There should be less than 2 RBCs per hpf.
- If three or more RBCs are present in multiple samples, it indicated the presence of microscopic hematuria.

Blood:

- Blood should not be present in urine.
- The presence of blood is referred to as hematuria, and warrants a proper workup of the patient to evaluate the cause.
- Various causes of hematuria are kidney stones, urinary tract infection, kidney disease such as glomerulonephritis, or malignancies.

Epithelial cells:

The urine specimen may contain squamous epithelial cells from the urethra, or transitional epithelial cells from the bladder.

There should be less than 15 to 20 cells per hpf.

This may be increased if the collected urine sample is contaminated.

Casts:

Casts are basically cylindrical particles formed by coagulated protein, which is secreted by the renal tubular cells. There are different types of casts that may be seen, and these are outlined in Box 2.

BOX 2. TYPES OF CASTS FOUND IN URINE SPECIMENS	
CAST TYPE	CONDITIONS THEY ARE FOUND
Hyaline casts	Healthy individuals (<5/hpf) Increased – strenuous exercise
Red cell casts	Glomerulonephritis Vasculitis
White cell casts	Tubulointerstitial nephritis Acute pyelonephritis Renal tuberculosis
Granular casts (muddy brown)	Acute tubular necrosis
Waxy casts/ broad casts	Advanced renal failure
Fatty casts (maltese -cross appearance)	Nephrotic syndrome

Crystals:

When the dissolved substances in urine take on a solid form, they are referred to as crystals.

Occasional crystals may be present normally, that form from normal urine solutes. Sometimes, however, crystals that are formed may be diagnostic of certain diseases. These are outlined in Box 3.

BOX 3. TYES OF CRYSTALS SEEN IN URINE SPECIMEN		
COMPOSITION	SHAPE	CONDITION THAT IT IS SEEN IN
Calcium oxalate	Envelope shaped	Ethylene glycol ingestion – acute kidney injury
Uric acid	Diamond or barrel shaped	Tumor lysis syndrome – acute kidney injury Gout
Cysteine	Hexagonal	Cysteinuria
Magnesium ammonium phosphate and triple phosphate	Coffin lid shaped	Urinary tract infections

Bacteria:

- No bacteria must be present in a normal urine sample.
- Presence of bacteria indicates either infection, or contamination of the specimen.
- If bacteria are present along with positive leukocyte esterase and nitrites, urinary tract infection must be suspected and must be correlated clinically.
- If however, squamous cells are alone increased, it is likely that the specimen is contaminated.
- If a urinary tract infection is suspected, the urine sample must be sent for culture and sensitivity.

Yeasts:

- A normal urine sample will not show presence of yeasts.
- Again, its presence signifies either infection or contamination of the specimen.

Volume: Normal lab value for volume is 800 – 2,500 mL in 24 hours.

STOOL ANALYSIS:

This test analyses fecal matter to diagnose problems related to the gastrointestinal system, and sometimes other systemic pathologies.

GROSS EXAMINATION:

- Normal stools are brown, formed or semi-formed. Infant stools may be yellow-green and semi formed. Change in consistency is seen in infective diarrhea.
- Gross examination may reveal presence of parasites like tapeworm, cysts, or trophozoites.

SCREENING TESTS:

Detection of blood in the stool (fecal occult blood test):

- Various causes of blood in the stool include carcinoma, hemorrhoids, Crohn's disease, or an ulcer in the GI tract.
- When it occurs in the upper GI tract, often the blood appears dark or black and when the bleeding is in the lower GI region, the blood is often red.

MICROBIOLOGICAL EXAMINATION:

- The stool sample is stained with methylene blue and mounted on a glass slide.
- Presence of pus cells indicates bacterial infection.

- o >50 pus cells per hpf along with macrophages and erythrocytes indicates shigellosis.
- o <20 pus cells per hpf may be seen in salmonellosis and E. coli infections.
- Hanging drop preparation may be used to view any motile organisms.
- Stool culture may also be done to isolate specific types of bacteria causing gastrointestinal infections.

CHEMICAL TESTS:

Stool pH:

- Normal stool pH is 7 to 7.5.
- A pH below 5.6 is characteristic of carbohydrate malabsorption.

Tests for steatorrhea:

- This measures the absorption of dietary fat.
- When fat is not absorbed, it is often the result of intestinal disease, pancreatic insufficiency, or bile duct obstruction.
- Indications for this test include:
  - o Reduced vitamin D absorption, which results in osteomalacia
  - o Decreased serum levels show lower carotene absorption

- o Low vitamin K absorption, which can result in hemorrhage
- This test quantitatively assesses a 72-hour stool specimen for fat. The interpretation is as follows:
  - o normal < 5g per day
  - o Equivocal 5 -7 g
  - o Steatorrhea > 7g
- Examination through a microscope of fat-stained stool smear is also done.
- Steatorrhoea can also be assessed by measuring the absorption of ^{125}I oleic acid and ^{131}I triolein. The pill containing both is administered orally. After 4 hours a blood specimen is tested.
  - o There is impaired pancreatic function when absorption of oleic acid is normal while triolein uptake is abnormal.
  - o Failure of absorption of both shows the malabsorption of the fat is not related to the pancreas – true steatorrhoea.

Test for reducing sugars:

- Stool sample is checked for lactose.
- This would be present in infants with lactase deficiency, who are therefore unable to convert lactose into glucose and galactose.
- This presents clinically as colic, and a failure to thrive, which indicates the presence of lactose intolerance.

Test for urobilinogen:

- Conjugated bilirubin from the liver is converted to urobilinogen, which is excreted from the body via urine and stools.
- Normal value excreted in stools: 50 – 300 mg/day
- This value decreases in biliary tract obstruction, liver disease, and oral antibiotic therapy.

Fecal osmotic gap:

- This calculates the concentration of electrolytes in stool.
- In secretory diarrhea, the osmotic gap is less than 50 mosm/kg.
- In osmotic diarrhea, the osmotic gap is more than 150 mosm/kg

CEREBROSPINAL FLUID ANALYSIS

Cerebrospinal fluid is produced in the choroid plexus of the ventricles of the brain. It provides mechanical cushioning to the brain, serves to transport metabolites and other compounds, and maintains homeostasis. Any patient who is suspected of having injury to the brain, or infection that may have extended to the brain, is subjected to CSF analysis. CSF analysis tests the following components:

Gross appearance:

- Normal CSF should be clear and colorless.
- Turbid/milky CSF: Infectious meningitis
- Xantochromic/colored CSF: Brain bleed, kernicterus, tumors like melanoma or melanosarcoma.
- Cloudy CSF: Associated with increased protein content, this is due to disorders of the blood-brain barrier.

Biochemistry:

The various components of CSF, and conditions in which their normal level changes are given below, in Box 3.

BOX 3: CSF BIOCHEMISTRY		
COMPONENT	NORMAL LEVEL	CHANGED IN
Glucose	45 – 80 mg/dl 60 – 80% of plasma	Decreases in meningitis
Lactate	< 20 – 25 mg/dl	Raised in intracranial hemorrhage, trauma, meningitis
Glutamine	8 – 18 mg/dl	Liver disease

		Reye syndrome
Albumin	500 times lower than serum	Damage to blood brain barrier -

Microscopic tests:

- Studying the CSF under a microscope may show the following findings:

- Lymphocytosis: Meningitis, neurocysticercosis, multiple sclerosis, Guillian Barre syndrome

- Monocytosis: Chronic meningitis, CNS malignancies, intracranial hemorrhage

- Increased neutrophils: acute meningitis, brain abscess, cerebral infarct, previous lumbar puncture

SYNOVIAL FLUID ANALYSIS

Synovial fluid, or joint fluid, is present in all the joints of the body and is an ultra-filtrate of blood plasma. Usually, its composition is also similar to that of plasma but it may change during inflammatory conditions of the joint. Synovial fluid evaluation is done under the following categories:

Physical examination:

- Appearance is clear.

- In non-inflammatory conditions, such as osteoarthritis and trauma, it may be yellow.
- Synovial fluid has a high viscosity which may decrease in arthritis.
- Inflammatory conditions change the color to dense yellow, with turbidity and crystal formation.
- Septic conditions may give the fluid a yellow green, cloudy appearance. Trauma to joint results in reddish fluid.

Chemical examination:

- Glucose: usually similar to blood glucose levels. This may be deceased in inflammatory conditions such as ankylosis, sepsis, and gout.
- Proteins: This is normally one-third of the levels present in serum. However, it may be increased in inflammatory and hemorrhagic disorders.

Microscopic analysis:

- Leukocyte count: This is usually less than 200 cells per μl.
- Neutrophils form less than 25% of these cells.
- Non-inflammatory conditions tend to raise the white blood cell count, but it is still less than 2000 cells per μl. It is further significantly increased in inflammation.

REFERENCES:

1. Post TW, Rose BD. Urinalysis in the diagnosis of renal disease. Curhan GC and Forman JP (Eds)

2. Urinalysis. Lab Tests Online. Available at http://labtestsonline.org/understanding/analytes/urinalysis/tab/sample. Accessed: 12/01/2018.

3. King Strasinger S, Schaub DiLorenzo M. *Urinalysis and Body Fluids Testing*. 5th ed. Philadelphia, PA: F.A. Davis; 177-199.

4. Anderson MJ, Agarwal R. Urinalysis. Lerma EV and Nissenson AR. *In Nephrology Secrets*. Third Edition. Elsevier Mosby: 2012

5. Mahindrakar, A. (2013). Routine stool examination. *Pediatric Infectious Disease*, 5(4), pp.187-188.

EXERCISES:

1. Which of the following is not a normal value for amount of urine collected in 24 hours?

    a. 500 ml

    b. 900 ml

    c. 1200 ml

    d. 1700 ml

2. In which of the following conditions does the urine appear dark black?

    a. Hemoglobinurea

    b. Alkaptonuria

    c. Phenylketonuria

    d. Tyrosinemia

3. All the following components of urine examination point to urinary tract infection, except:

    a. Leukocyte esterase

    b. Nitrite

    c. Squamous cells

    d. Bacteria in urine

4. Which of the following conditions is not associated with occult blood in stools?

    a. Hemorrhoids

b. Colon cancer

c. Diarrhea

d. Gastric ulcers

5. If the stool examination shows that the patient has steartorrhoea, absorption of which of the following vitamins is not affected?

 a. Vitamin A

 b. Vitamin C

 c. Vitamin D

 d. Vitamin K

14. APPENDIX I: THERAPEUTIC MEDICATION LEVELS

These tests check for the levels of medicine present in the blood. When the blood has a certain level of a drug, it becomes effective to treat the medical condition. This type of test is required for patients who take the following drugs:

- Antibiotics like gentamicin to treat infections
- Phenytoin to treat seizures
- Digoxin to treat abnormal heart beats

Here are the normal lab values for some drugs that people take.

- Amikacin: 15 to 25 mcg/mL
- Aminophylline: 10 to 20 mcg/mL
- Amitriptyline: 120 to 150 ng/mL
- Carbamazepine: 5 to 12 mcg/mL
- Cyclosporine: 100 to 400 ng/mL (12 hours after dose)
- Desipramine: 150 to 300 ng/mL
- Digoxin: 0.8 to 2.0 ng/mL
- Disopyramide: 2 to 5 mcg/mL
- Ethosuximide: 40 to 100 mcg/mL
- Flecainide: 0.2 to 1.0 mcg/mL
- Gentamicin: 5 to 10 mcg/mL
- Imipramine: 150 to 300 ng/mL
- Kanamycin: 20 to 25 mcg/mL
- Lithium: 0.8 to 1.2 mEq/L
- Nortriptyline: 50 to 150 ng/mL
- Phenobarbital: 10 to 30 mcg/mL
- Phenytoin: 10 to 20 mcg/mL
- Primidone: 5 to 12 mcg/mL
- Procainamide: 4 to 10 mcg/mL
- Quinidine: 2 to 5 mcg/mL
- Salicylate: varies with dosage
- Sirolimus: 4 to 20 ng/mL (12 hours after dose; varies with use)

- Tacrolimus: 5 to 15 ng/mL (12 hours after dose)

- Theophylline: 10 to 20 mcg/mL

- Tobramycin: 5 to 10 mcg/mL

Note:

- *mcg/mL = microgram per milliliter*

- *ng/mL = nanogram per milliliter*

- *mEq/L = milliequivalents per liter*

- *mcmol = micromole*

15. APPENDIX II: TEST PANELS FOR VARIOUS CLINICAL SITUATIONS

A set of laboratory tests that are grouped together is referred to as a panel. The panel may be composed of tests intended to diagnose a specific disease, or else may be based on the type of specimen provided.

BASIC METABOLIC PANEL:

- It is also called CHEM-7 or SMA-7 (Sequential Multiple Analysis)
- This test is done when it is necessary to diagnose acute medical conditions, which would require immediate management.

The components are:

COMPONENT ASSESSED	TO DIAGNOSE
Four electrolytes: Sodium Potassium Chloride Bicarbonate	Dehydration Water intoxication Acid-base disorders
Blood Urea Nitrogen	Renal or liver failure
Creatinine	Renal failure
Glucose	Hypoglycemic shock/ hyperglycemic ketoacidosis

COMPREHENSIVE METABOLIC PANEL:

The CMP is a set of 14 tests that includes the BMP and information on blood proteins and liver. This includes the following tests:

- Albumin
- Blood urea nitrogen (BUN)
- Calcium

- Carbon dioxide (Bicarbonate)
- Chloride
- Creatinine
- Glucose
- Potassium
- Sodium
- Total Bilirubin
- Total Protein
- Alanine aminotransferase (ALT)
- Alkaline phosphatase (ALP)
- Aspartate aminotransferase (AST)

ROUTINE BLOOD TEST PANEL:

This is done for annual medical examinations. It serves as a screen to detect underlying problems, and, if found abnormal, further investigations can be done. This panel includes:

- Complete blood count: Hemogram
- Blood chemistry:
    - Glucose
    - Urea,
    - BUN
    - Creatinine
    - Liver function tests
    - Lipid profile
- Routine Urine Analysis

PRE-SURGICAL PANEL:

This panel is routinely done prior to surgery in order to detect any systemic pathologies that might be affected by anesthesia and surgery. It also serves to detect infections that might prompt the surgical team to observe universal precautions. This panel includes the following tests:

- Complete blood count
- Blood chemistry:
    - o Glucose
    - o BUN
    - o Creatinine
- Serological tests:
    - o HIV I and II
    - o HBsAg
- Routine Urine analysis.
- Chest X-ray and electrocardiogram are also taken.
- In selected cases with positive history, the following are also performed:
    - o Liver function tests
    - o Electrocardiogram
    - o Thyroid function tests

16. CONCLUSION

Now that we have learned about the various laboratory values and their clinical significance, it is important to recognize that, although these laboratory values have an important role to play in the diagnosis and management of patients, they are, at the end of the day, only an adjunct to the larger sphere of the patients' case history and clinical examination. Even if a certain laboratory test has returned back as 'normal', the patient must be examined for clinically relevant signs and symptoms. On the other hand, if the test results are abnormal, the patient must be definitely examined for correlating signs and symptoms, and this examination must be repeated periodically for checking improvement or worsening of the patients' condition. Similarly, serial laboratory tests must be assessed for 'trending'.

It is important to remember that the laboratory values section of the NCLEX and other exams do not merely test the numbers in the various ranges of laboratory tests. The idea is to test whether the student is capable of recognizing an abnormal result, and, once recognized, whether the student has enough knowledge to act on the abnormal result. Therefore, questions in this section will not just be about normal ranges of laboratory values, it will also have questions related to analysis and application. Of course, all students need to be aware of the normal ranges too, and many students have doubts in this area, as normal laboratory values tend to differ slightly with each healthcare facility. However, the these exams do not expect you to memorize each and every value, any 'out of range' value given will be far away from the normal range.

We hope you enjoyed reading and learning from this book. It gives you insight into how to prepare the correct way. Only if you prepare well, will you succeed.

Wish you success in your medical career!

17. ANSWERS TO EXERCISES

CHAPTER I

1. a

2. c

3. b

4. b

5. d

CHAPTER II

1. a

2. b

3. c

4. b

5. a

6. d

7. b

8. b

9. b

10. b

11. d

CHAPTER III

1. d

2. b

3. c

4. d

5. d

CHAPTER IV

1. d

2. a

3. b

4. b

5. a

CHAPTER V

1. d

2. b

3. a

4. d

5. b

CHAPTER VI

1. d

2. d

3. b

4. a

5. b

CHAPTER VII

1. b

2. d

3. a

4. c

5. c

CHAPTER VIII

1. c

2. b

3. a

4. b

5. c

CHAPTER IX

1. b

2. b

3. a

4. d

5. d

CHAPTER X

1. d

2. b

3. c

4. a

5. c

CHAPTER XI

1. c

2. b

3. c

4. c

5. b

CHAPTER XII

1. a

2. b

3. c

4. c

5. b

JOIN OUR COMMUNITY

Medical Creations is an educational company focused on providing study tools for Healthcare students.

We want to be as close as possible to our customers, that's why we are active on all the main Social Media platforms.

You can find us here:

Facebook **www.facebook.com/medicalcreations**

Instagram **www.instagram.com/medicalcreations**

Twitter **www.twitter.com/medicalcreation** (no 's')

Pinterest **www.pinterest.com/medicalcreations**

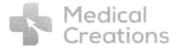

LAB VALUES

CHECK OUT OUR OTHER BOOKS

BEST SELLER ON AMAZON:

Medical Terminology:

The Best and Most Effective Way to Memorize, Pronounce and Understand Medical Terms

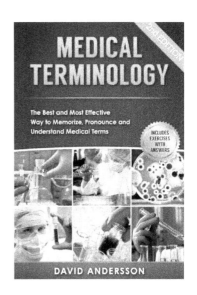

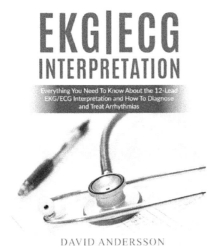

BEST SELLER ON AMAZON:

EKG/ECG Interpretation: Everything you Need to Know about the 12-Lead ECG/EKG Interpretation and How to Diagnose and Treat Arrhythmias

www.ingramcontent.com/pod-product-compliance
Lightning Source LLC
LaVergne TN
LVHW020338080725
815534LV00001B/71